Caregiving: *Our* Labor *of* Love

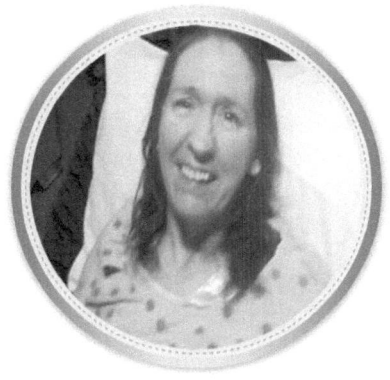

A MEMOIR

John Patterson

Volume One

Inspiring Voices

Inspiring Voices books may be ordered through booksellers or by contacting:

Inspiring Voices
1663 Liberty Drive
Bloomington, IN 47403
www.inspiringvoices.com
1 (866) 697-5313

ISBN: 978-1-4624-1137-5 (sc)
ISBN: 978-1-4624-1138-2 (e)

Library of Congress Control Number: 2015910451

Print information available on the last page.

Inspiring Voices rev. date: 5/3/2016

To the reader:

Introduction

My name is John Patterson and this book is about the successful caregiving experience I gained while caregiving for my wife Sue Ann Patterson from March 2007 to September of 2013. I hope you can find how a person who is caring for a family member can do the right things to bring about blessings from the Lord as you go down this path that has been given to you. I hope to show you not only better ways but blessed ways through our story. May you see God in our story for He was in our midst and blessings came to us daily. Since, one has to take it day by day in caregiving.

There are things in this book that will bless you from day one to the end of the caregiving experience. Caregiving is wrought with hurdles which provide unrelenting pressures from both Society and family. Transitioning into caregiving is not smooth to say the least. There are huge mountains and low valleys that both the caring person and the one who is receiving care will have to experience.

My daughter Jennifer said to me,

"I wished seven years ago someone would have set me down and told me what to expect these last seven years."

Through this painful battle my family and I experienced we hope to provide you with the tools needed to survive that battle. So you know how to care, and combat the hard-hitting times. So you can find the passion for caring that a minority of people only will experience in their lifetimes. I did not know what I was getting into when I found myself becoming a caregiver. For caregiving is much like a flood. It begins as a trickle signifying the slow embodied changes of a thriving person. Before realizing it the trickle bursts into a downward spiral leaving you to only ponder what life once was.

I wrote this book due to my disheartening realization that I had no reference to turn to for peace of mind. Every day marked a new threshold and chipped away a little more. There was no where I could turn to for information that I so desperately desired. Information is the key to making a difference and lightening a significant load. Far too many of us have gone before you struggling day after day. I hope that you will find that there is so much information in this book that you can have an easier time with caring. Caring is not easy; in fact it is at times seems impossible!

I am writing this introduction just three days after Sue passed away. It is an amazingly unbelievable story we lived through and this book comes from my heart and Soul. I have peace in my heart and Soul for I know I did my best for Sue. I have no regrets for the process molded and shaped me into a better person and a better man of God. I feel we went through the fire and came out purer on the other side of caregiving.

In addition to the stresses of caregiving I was at many times shocked by what I found in research. I stumbled upon an article online from the National Center for Biotechnology. The article was written as Advances in Patient Safety. It was a study of patient's safety in the home. What caught my eye was this sentence,

"Home health care is the fastest growing sector in the health care industry, with an anticipated growth of 66 percent over the next 10 years and with over 7 million patients served each year."

Seven million people and their caregivers are going to be in the same situation Sue and I stumbled into. Seventy million Souls in ten years will be in the home caring situation that our family has experienced. For more information, go to http://ncbi.nlm.nih.gov/books.NBK43619/ on the web.

I could not place Sue into a Nursing home due to our income and yet I could not do much due to the huge expense of caring in the home. I will show you how to transition from a conventional standpoint to a life centered on your caregiving.

Regardless of my reasons the most important underlining issue is a bid for change. I write this book praying that a revolution in the healthcare system may one day be enacted. We need change on the Federal, State and County level. I suffered from an astounding $20,507 in tax deductions in 2010. Our lives became controlled by our finances. We lived based on a fixed income of my salary as a Correctional Officer, and Sue's disability checks. Despite the staggering cost of in home care I was disregarded for any type of assistance from the limited programs established to help persons such as us. The only assistance I received from any Government program was a ramp for my home to go from my home to the street from Texas Department of Assistive Rehabilitation (DARS). Outside of DARS we received no help from any other Government services.

Since no other assistance came from the Federal Government, State of Texas, or County of residence. I reached new resolve that if our government would not help then God would supply my only solace. If you are called into caregiving then God shall provide for you and your needs. Thus let us begin our story that will hopefully bless you in the coming days, months, and years as you take on the revered work of caregiving.

(Please note if you are in caregiving or about to go into caregiving take a highlighter or pen and make notes as you read with concepts that you may put into practice).

Prologue

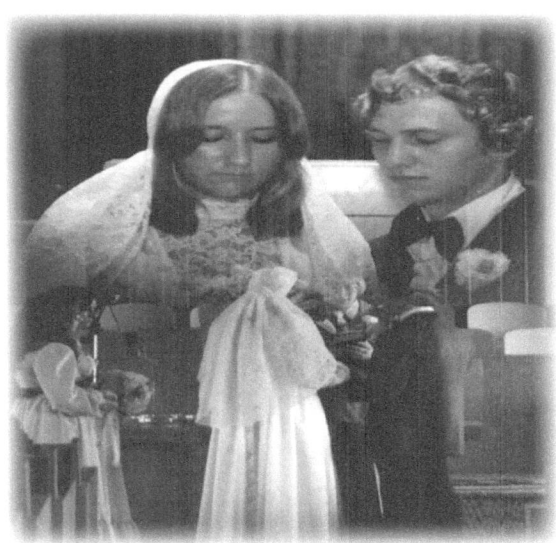

In April of 1981 a coworker and I traveled from Missouri to Arkansas for a weekend canoe trip. My wife Sue, and I were recently separated and I needed some kind of stress reliever. We camped out overnight on our trip, and early the next morning began unpacking supplies and the canoe.

We began placing the canoe into the river when I heard a rather frantic voice shouting from atop the hill.

"Are you John Patterson?" The man called out.

"Yes I am." I replied.

The man continued frantically calling my name as he slid down the hill in an effort to reach me.

.

"Here, you need to call this number immediately." He said handing me a piece of paper.

I looked down at the piece of paper and remotely listened as the man ushered me towards his house a short distance away which contained a telephone. I was not sure what was going on or who this man was.

We scurried towards his home, my thoughts racing wildly. I twiddled the paper in my hands while placing the phone call to a number I recognized as my employer's. Time slowed to a screeching halt while I waited, and waited as the phone rang in what actually was only a few seconds.

"Thank you for calling Skaggs, how may I help you?" A familiar voice chirped.

"This is John Patterson. I have an urgent message from someone there."

"Hold for a minute please."

Several moments passed as I continued to wait for someone to answer. I scoured my brain to try and think of a plausible explanation for such a bizarre encounter. Why would my employer call me unless it was pressing?

"John, whatever you're doing stop it. Get back home now." My supervisor blurted ending the deadening silence.

"What's going on?" I asked.

"I cannot tell you right now. Just get back home now."

Several minutes passed of our back and forth banter while I demanded answers. It became apparent and evident I would get none until I was back in Springfield, Missouri. I hung up the phone and racked my brain for possibilities while we traveled down the hill to the river to reload the car, and start the seven hour drive home. I was a twenty one-year-old kid who had never experience any life altering event before; needless to say I was naïve of the possibilities.

Several hours into the drive around Branson, Missouri a news report beckoned from the radio.

"A tragic accident has left many in Springfield, Missouri speechless following an incident of drunk driving late last night. A drunk driver ran a red light at the intersection of Division Street, and Kansas Expressway. There is currently one possible fatality; names are being withheld pending notification of the next of kin. We will bring you any updates as they develop."

I kneeled over in the seat, feeling as if the wind was knocked out of me.

"Oh my God, It's Sue, it has to be Sue." I said looking towards my coworker.

"How do you know that, they didn't give a name?"

"I know it in my Soul, I can feel it." I said.

CHAPTER ONE

The Praying Days

James 5:16 (KJV) "Confess your faults one to another, and pray one for another, that ye may be healed. The effectual fervent prayer of a righteous man availed much."

I peered over Sue's shoulder one January night in 2004. I discovered Sue was visiting Guideposts website.

"What are you doing?" I asked.

"I am putting in a prayer." She said.

"What do you mean you're putting in a prayer?" I asked.

"I put in a prayer need, then it asks for my email address and then I click send. It goes to Guideposts server site and then trained volunteer reads my prayer request and lifts my request up in prayer and then sends that prayer written especially for me back to my email box." She said.

I was intrigued from the moment Sue told me, and immediately wanted to delve deeper into their ministry. The next day I called to the Guideposts headquarters and inquired about their organization. We discussed my status as an Ordained Minister, and that I wanted more information on the organization. Later that day I faxed a copy of my ordination so that I could begin the involvement process. Almost instantaneously, I was in it head first and I was praying for people like Sue.

The years of my involvement with Guideposts reaped of blessings, and I basked in the power of prayer. With my employment with the State of Texas I generally work an average of a six days work rotation with three days off. This provided me with one full day committed purely to prayer. My involvement consisted of volunteering with the Personal Prayer Response (PPR's).

I would often attack the prayer board, praying all day until the prayer requests went to zero. One day Mary Ann Gillespie from Guideposts called me.

"We have a good problem." She said.

"What's the problem?" I asked.

"You are praying up all the prayers on the board. The average volunteer does thirty five prayers a month. You are doing thirty five prayers a day. We have many people who are new volunteers and they are not getting the experience that they need to due to you are praying up all the prayers on the board. We need you to back off a little." She said.

I laughed but felt the wisdom that Mary Ann was saying to me. So I reduced the PPR's and transitioned into prayer via the phone for Guideposts. Their phone ministry consisted of a volunteer calling the Guidepost server and entering their telephone number. Those in need of prayer would call the number listed and then be connected to a volunteer like myself. I found this more challenging as it was much more personal than PPR's. Shortly thereafter I found myself logging into the phone and going online to the PPR's at the same time. When I received a phone call I would stop the online prayers for a moment, pray with the person on the phone and return to the computer.

In September of 2005 I received a call from Rev. Dr. Peola Hicks, the manager of Guideposts. "With all the prayers you are doing we have decided to make you our Volunteer of the Year." She said.

Sue and I were thrilled and immediately began planning for our impending trip. Initially the Guideposts donor conference was scheduled towards the end of the month in Houston, Texas. However, as luck would have it Nature had a different idea and the Houston area was devastated by *Hurricane Rita*. We watched from our house that was located near the interstate connecting Houston to Dallas as thousands upon thousands of people fled the Houston area. The interstate was littered with Souls trying to escape the chaos. Soon cars began to clog the interstate and we realized that many people were running out of gas while their cars sat idly not moving for hours. The gas stations around us soon ran out of gas as well. It quickly became clear that the conference was cancelled and we would not be going anywhere anytime soon.

Later on that year Peola called to inform us of the change of venue. She told us that the conference was changed to Phoenix, Arizona and that courtesy of Guideposts we would be receiving airfare and hotel expense for the trip. To our surprise Sue and I were ushered to the Hilton Hotel. On the day of our visit we attended the fundraiser where I was called in front of the crowd and presented with the Volunteer of the Year Award. The plaque was beautiful and I was humbled to have been part of the event.

One day Mary Ann Gillespie from Guidepost calls me and informs me of a new prayer program, Real Time Prayer, © Live Person, Inc. 2014, that uses instant messaging software that enables the prayer volunteer and person requesting prayer to "meet" online for prayer in real time. I soon found myself sitting in my home at my computer praying with people from all over the world with the touch of a few keystrokes. Shortly after this new live program, I found myself yet again upping the ante with prayer. I was logging onto the phones, logging onto Live Person, and going to the PPR's at the same time. I began my day of prayer at 7 A.M and finished at 10 P.M. During this process I felt a persistent and beautiful change for the better.

I kept praying away throughout 2005. At some point in 2006 I received a phone call from Guidepost. They invited me to participate in a volunteer video. I was whole-heartedly eager to participate in the video, hopeful that it would touch someone's life. They filmed the video at three different locations. Included in the video was a woman named Mary from Ohio, a church in South Dallas, and lastly mine and Sue's home. I was slated to present information to the viewer regarding PPR's. Sue participated in the making of the video but is only visible for a few seconds.

Shortly before completion at our house I remember quiet clearly speaking with the lead production member. "Your home is a Fortress," he said in reference to the rock solidness of our Spirituality. As if nothing and no one could penetrate the solidity of our life. Sue and I were at that time gratified.

I had a flat tire ministry during this time. As I ran to town and back I would find an assortment of different types of people, all who were stuck on the side of the road with a flat tire. I would pull over and ask them if they wanted my help, most said, "Yes" so I would get their spare out and change the tire. It came to a point that I would ask some if they believed in the power of prayer. If they said, "Yes" I would ask them to pray for us. When I prayed online I would ask people from all over the world to pray for us there as well.

Life was going well and thriving spiritually for me. Shortly thereafter is when life took a turn for the worse and I realized nothing would ever be as simple as before. I was about to begin the biggest test of my Faith. Caregiving!

Guidepost, *OurPrayer* service is the part of their services that I was part of in them blessed years. I would say that their mission that follows was a success in me:

Faith, Hope, and the Power of Prayer

Guideposts offer tools and services that empower individuals to deepen their relationship with God and with others through the power of prayer. *OurPrayer* is a community of faith comforting people through prayer. We're here when you need us: You may submit a prayer request via our website, 24x7. Guideposts receive over a million prayer requests a year. Answered Prayers are testimonials of the power of prayer at work. Join us to pray for others who submit prayer requests online.

For more information for Guidepost go to:

http://www.guideposts.org/about-us

CHAPTER TWO

The Commitment

In March of 2007, Sue, Jennifer and I were spending what we thought was a normal day like any other together. Sue was in front of the computer, and Jennifer was not so surprisingly watching television like a typical teenager. At some point Sue turned to us and began to talk with slurred speech. Jennifer approached her, peering down at the corner of her mouth; the left side of her mouth seemed to droop and did not appear to be functioning at the same pace as her right side.

"Dad, this looks like a stroke. It looks like she had a stroke!" Jennifer said somewhat frantically.

"Sue, what's wrong with you? Maybe it is a stroke," I said.

Sue looked back and forth between the two of us, shrugging. Clearly none of us knew and were merely guessing. I immediately called a Neurologist, and we headed to Dallas later that day. Initially the doctors informed us that Sue had two frontal lobe strokes. The left side of her body was affected as well. We came home, and I immediately flashed back to 1981.

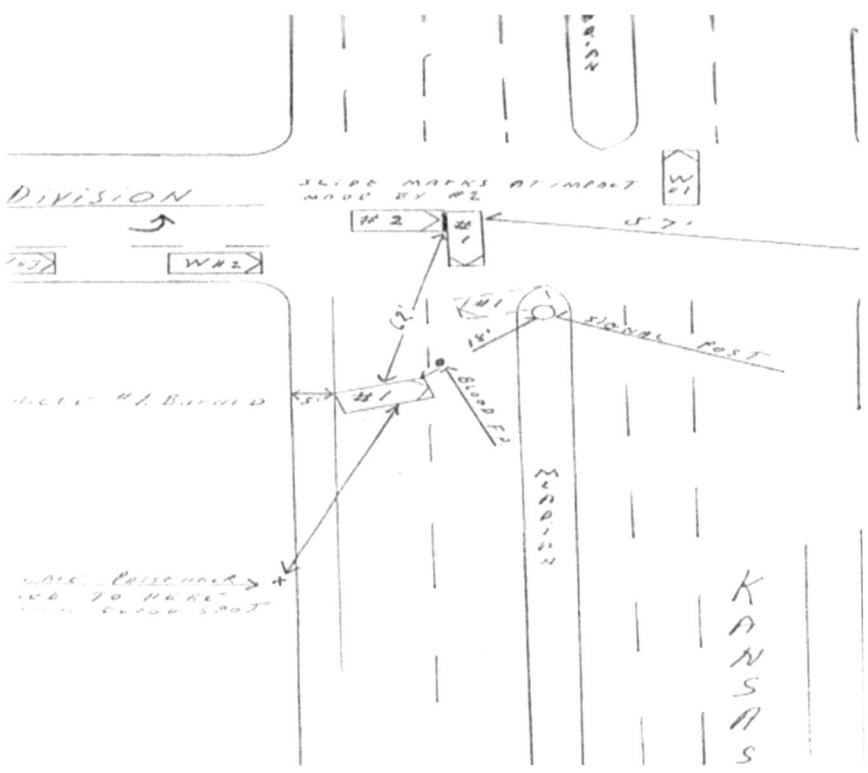

I felt myself retracing the steps from so many years ago when I had gotten down upon my knees, asking God to save my wife.

The first stop I made after returning from the canoe trip was to my apartment. I found taped to my apartment door a scribbled note from a police officer:

Mr. Patterson you need to go to Cox Medical
North to find your wife Sue Patterson.

I immediately had my friend drive me to the hospital and was directed by nursing staff to her room in an intensive care unit (ICU). I entered the room and thought there was a mistake, this person did not look like my wife for she looked like a stranger to me that I did not recognize. I smelt the overpowering stench of dead flesh of her body. Looking down at her body lying in the hospital bed I tried to see past the burns covering her left side, trailing from her feet to her head which had swollen larger than a basketball.

I didn't notice as the three doctors entered the room, the shock of what laid before me was raw, and unforgiving. They began talking amongst themselves before turning their attention toward me.

"Mr. Patterson?" The first doctor asked. I nodded slowly attempting to listen while staring at my wife.

"Due to her swelling on the brain she will most likely become non-responsive vegetated state for she has severe brain damage." The first doctor said.

"The injury to her flesh from the burns will most likely lead to an infection, which will be fatal." The second doctor said.

"She will most likely never awaken from the coma." The third doctor said.

I thanked the doctors very briefly for their medical opinions, and for what they were doing for Sue. The exchange was rather brief but I imagined they realized I was struggling to process what I was witnessing before me.

I walked to a phone booth and attempted to call Sue's mother Flora, who had not yet been notified. I struggled to speak, and every time I blubbered out what was happening gibberish escaped my mouth. I finally hung up unable to perform a basic interaction. I walked around aimlessly in the hospital before finding myself at the chapel; I dropped to my knees and pleaded for God to save my wife. Hours later after regaining my composure I was able to alert Flora to Sue's plight.

Our two-year-old son, Travis was in the car with Sue. He was pulled to safety from the flaming vehicle and had obtained minor burns to his buttocks. I was directed to his room which was on a

8

different floor of the same hospital. I held him, and hugged him before leaving the hospital.

I borrowed a car and drove to my apartment and packed everything as fast as I could before driving to the apartment Sue, and I had once shared. I opened the door just wide enough to throw everything I packed up into the car with all my belonging through the door way before returning to the hospital to stay indefinitely.

I learned at the hospital that Sue and Travis were traveling in our car when they were hit by the drunk driver who was identified as our neighbor. Sue was thrown from the car and had broken the C2 vertebrae of her neck (the same vertebrae broken by Christopher Reeves). While lying in the street gasoline trickled from the tank of the car to her body and ignited. Over forty percent of her body was engulfed by flames, and Travis was pulled from the car. Sue initially died at the scene, and was encircled by a group of by standers who pulled her from the fire and began praying for her. Once the ambulance arrived she was revived and rushed to the hospital approximately two blocks from the accident.

I veraciously prayed over the course of a month for Sue to awaken from her coma. Based on what the doctor told me I became obsessed with seeing her wake up. I thought the hardest part of her recovery would be her coma ending, and that we would be out of the woods once she attained consciousness. I immediately realized the mistake of my prayer when she awoke to a painful nightmare. "Oh my God my body hurts!" She screamed out in tremendous pain as I witnessed Sue place a towel between her teeth and gnash her teeth in agony, almost cutting the towel into two pieces due to the pain from her burns.

Once Sue awoke her treatment began, the course of her treatment caused Sue the most brutal experience I have ever witnessed in my life. Specialty burn units did not exist yet, and the treatment for burns was done on regular hospital floors. Sue was placed in a one hundred gallon tank of hot water, and left to soak for half an hour before having her dead skin pulled away by nurses. A treatment known as Debridement, Sue experienced these treatments several times.

After the Debridement was deemed successful she was given skin grafts. Skin was taken from her right thigh, and run through a mesh machine to stretch the skin, leaving the skin with the appearance of fish net panty hose, before being placed on the exposed area of what was once burnt flesh. After the skin grafts were completed her neck brace was removed and a halo was surgically screwed into her skull in order to stabilize her neck, and fuse her vertebrae. A bone was taken from her hip, and was wired and screwed to her vertebrae. Several months later she began to sit up well enough to sit comfortably in a wheelchair. I began taking her on tours of the hospital, and short lived trips outside to get her out of the room she was constantly confined to other then when in operating rooms.

One day we were having our usual afternoon stroll when I saw a sign dictating a section of the hospital as the *City Hospital*.

"Oh Sue, let's go see what in the *City Hospital*." I said to her.

Sue gave a thumb up in agreement as I pushed open the double doors and we entered. I looked around and quickly realized it was the hospital morgue. I immediately did an about-face and swiveled the wheelchair around.

"Let's get out of here!!" I exclaimed.

Sue began laughing uncontrollably as we retreated to a safe place. Over the course of our continued hospital captivity Sue continued to make small progress. She started reading the Dictionary in determination to relearn her vocabulary, and ultimately speak again. In her road of recovery she had to relearn how to talk and walk again.

I needed to get back to work for I had taken off over two and one half months just being by Sue's side in the hospital. I was drained and exhausted. We lived in the North side of town in Springfield, Missouri and I worked on the South East side of town. So I started out early that morning in the dark walking the ten miles or so just to get to work. I noticed there was no cars on this highway under construction so I went down that road thinking it would be safer since no traffic was allowed in that area. I was walking along and for some reason I looked down at my feet just in time to stop! I was on the edge of a fifty foot drop off. They were building a bridge and it was not completed yet but in the dark I could not see that. I almost died that morning. After that day, I got an old bicycle and wore it out going to work until I could afford a car again.

I continued to beg God to heal Sue. Over the next ten years, Sue made a complete recovery, baffling doctors. She experienced more heartache and pain than most could ever imagine. Sue finally, was able to live a normal life again; she gave birth to our second and last child, Jennifer, in 1988. We survived the nightmare and moved forward with our lives. In fact God had healed Sue so well that we would have conflict with someone every time we parked in a handicap parking area up front of the stores. People would come up to us all the time as we got out of the car. "You cannot park there that for handicap people," they would say.

"Call the police John they are harassing us," Sue would demand. Then one day we had enough and another man came up to us one night as we parked in the handicap parking area.

"You cannot park there," the man said.

"John I am calling the police," Sue said.

She did call the police and here they came. The man was still there bothering us when the police pulled up. We showed the police the sign that was register in the car window. Then we showed Sue's driver license that matched up with the sign in the car.

"Leave this couple alone or the next time they call us we will arrest you for harassment," The police told this man. I thought to myself,

Thank God for healing Sue so well we have to fight for a parking area where no one thinks she is disabled.

I thought those days were going to be the most horrific chapters of our lives, and that we could move forward in life. Thousands of dollars later, and countless surgeries we could be ordinary people again. Lightning as they say never strikes twice, or does it?

A new nightmare had begun—a different and evolved nightmare. I begged God to heal Sue as He had in 1981. I begged to be granted with a second unbelievable medical miracle. After I got on my knees and prayed, a few days later, all the effects of Sue's stroke were gone. Both sides of her mouth returned to normal. I praised God and thanked Him for granting my prayer. No sooner had I said that than the symptoms reappeared, from there it only seemed to intensify.

I was at work one day while Sue remained at home. Our routine was no different as she had maintained her status as a stay-at-home mom due to her lingering disability associated with the 1981 car wreck. Due to the nature of my employment as a Correctional Officer, contact with the world outside of the prison can be difficult, to say the least. On this particular day, Sue called the prison and managed to reach me.

"I am standing outside of the door of our house, and I cannot get back in," she said.

"Did you lock yourself out of the house?" I replied, puzzled at first by the conversation.

"No," she said.

I immediately reached out to my supervisor with concern, requesting to leave for a short period of time. We lived approximately thirty miles away from the prison. I rushed home to find Sue in the house already. I made sure she was settled in before returning to work, thinking the incident was of some minor concern. A few days later on my day off, we sat at the table for breakfast.

"No matter what, I want you to know I will be there for you. I committed to you the day we exchanged vows, and I will always love you dearly," I told her.

"I love you John," Sue said to me.

"I love you too honey," I replied to her.

I knew from that moment, based on the look on her face, she knew I would never abandon or mistreat her. I loved my wife dearly but was unaware of the hardship that was about to come upon us. I did not know the heart-wrenching brokenness of the gut-wrenching decision I had just made. I did commit to Sue because I loved her. We had been married since the late '70s. Later on it was that commitment that held us together, some days all we had was that commitment.

Days grew into weeks, which turned into months of a never-ending nightmare. Returning home from work each night felt as though I was coming home to a night shift at work. Only I never had any training in this new field. Caring for Sue was quickly turning into a crash course as I was thrown into it. My nightly routine would begin by assessing Sue. As I would walk through the door, I would look to see if any new symptoms had appeared. With each new symptom I would provide the doctors, the puzzle of what she was suffering from only magnified. It was an eerie feeling to see a symptom appear and disappear, followed by more starkly contrasted symptoms.

Sue began to complain about having a vertigo-like ailment where she felt dizzy constantly. She was still attempting to both care for herself and maintain a sense of independence, so much so she was still attempting to drive without even realizing how disastrous it could be.

"Jennifer, I need you to go to the store," Sue stated.

"Why?" asked Jennifer.

"I don't think I should drive anymore." Sue said matter-of-factly.

"What are you talking about?"

"Well I went to grocery store yesterday, and I guess I was all over the road, because a cop pulled me over," said Sue.

"What? Did you get a ticket or something?"

"No, he just thought I was drunk and pulled me over." Sue said.

It was the last time Sue attempted to drive and the last time she spoke of it. Her dizzy spells and headaches quickly turned from annoying to dangerous. She began to fall around the house, sometimes a couple of times a day. She became very stubborn, even while I was home, in an attempt to complete everyday activities. We lived in a small three bedroom mobile home that at the time allotted us the freedom to move. It swiftly however, began to feel like a prison busting at the seams. Out of fear for her safety, I soon purchased a shed and moved a vast majority of useless items from the house to the shed in an attempt to prevent objects from being in the way to trip her or hurt her if she did fall.

The shed that I purchased was rent to own. A Mennonites man drove up to our home with the shed on a trailer. I showed him where I wanted the shed. I started talking to him about his Brotherhood out of curiosity. I asked him about what God was doing in my life and how they would view my ministries?

"They would not let us do what you are doing on our own. We are a Brotherhood and the elders would have a say in what we do. We work as a community." He said.

I told him that I respected his life and The Brotherhood. I had this man back his trailer up and put the shed close to the house. The shed being so close to the house infuriated Sue. "John do not let him put that shed there!" Several years prior we planted a crape merle and the shed butted up so close that it bent the tree a bit. I got Sue to calm down and started packing up all the stuff that was or would be in the way of her falling. One of Sue's sisters tried to help us.

Sue's sister, Yvonne, a Licensed Practical Nurse (LPN), alarmed by her rapid descent from symptoms made the suggestion of purchasing Life Alert to give us the added security of knowing help was the push of a button away. Life Alert is a company that provides the purchaser a necklace that has a push button that when pushed alerts medical personnel to your location. Yvonne purchased it for us, and I thought maybe I could finally breathe a sigh of relief while at work. But of course, yet again I was wrong.

Attempting to use Life Alert was like attempting to put a Band-Aid on a severed artery. It did nothing to help prevent the falls, and there were too many falls occurring. We were attempting to use the service in a way that it was not meant to be used. She pushed the button while I was at work, and help came in the form of police kicking the front door down. When I returned from work, she was laying in our water bed, which she had difficulty laying in, when instead she should have been in the hospital bed. I had no option but to miss work and replace our door frame to secure our home.

The symptoms of the strokes led doctors to perform a Spinal Tap and MRI. Each trip to a doctor or hospital turned into a cycle in which Sue was poked and prodded often in painful ways. Results from tests gave doctors the impression that she was suffering from an assortment of possible illnesses. Whenever I noticed something new or unexpected it led doctors running down a new path. When her facial paralysis doctors steered her diagnosis to Strokes, or her hand shook it must be Parkinson's. Diseases began to intermingle in ways I had no idea was possible; according to the doctors she had two or three diseases that all became apparent at relatively the same time. All in all Sue was tested for the rarest of the rarest diseases and illnesses, some of which neither of us had ever heard of, such as CADASIL. CADASIL is a chromosomal disease in which a gene in one of the chromosome is bad. With the test for the disease being negative, doctors also speculated that she had perhaps been poisoned or come in contact with something environmentally. Speculation was all we were given, it was the only constant given to us by modern medicine. I Google CADASIL and here is the illness I believed Sue actually had.

What is CADASIL?

CADASIL (Cerebral Autosomal Dominant Arteriopathy with Sub-cortical Infarcts and Leukoencephalopathy) is an inherited form of cerebrovascular disease that occurs when the thickening of blood vessel walls blocks the flow of blood to the brain. The disease primarily affects small blood vessels in the white matter of the brain. A mutation in the Notch3 gene alters the muscular walls in these small arteries. CADASIL is characterized by migraine headaches and multiple strokes progressing to dementia. Other symptoms include cognitive deterioration, seizures, vision problems, and psychiatric problems such as severe depression and changes in behavior and personality. Individuals may also be at higher risk of heart attack. Symptoms and disease onset vary widely, with signs typically appearing in the mid-30s. Some individuals may not show signs of the disease until later in life. CADASIL — formerly known by several names, including hereditary multi-infarct dementia — is one cause of vascular cognitive impairment (dementia caused by lack of blood to several areas of the brain). It is an autosomal dominant inheritance disorder, meaning that one parent carries and passes on the defective gene. Most individuals with CADASIL have a family history of the disorder. However, because the genetic test for CADASIL was not available before 2000, many cases were misdiagnosed as multiple sclerosis, Alzheimer's disease, or other neurodegenerative diseases. For more information on CADASIL go to this web address:

http://www.ninds.nih.gov/disorders/cadasil/CADASIL.htm

Sue had two of these expensive tests done for CADASIL and she was negative on both tests. The test has false negatives results but no false positives results. Without having a proper diagnosis, it left us without any form of treatment. One night between Sue's pain and ongoing symptoms, I took her to the emergency room. I will never forget this night as we went to a hospital. We sat there for hours, and then the nurse came in and led us to a back room where he said, "This is the second waiting room." Wow he was not kidding and we found us waiting for couple more hours before a Doctor appeared, and his words resonated a truth I had not yet realized.

"There is absolutely nothing I can do for you. Here is a prescription for some pain medication, but that is all I can do." He said.

I began to realize there is no hospital where you can take someone suffering from a Neurological illness, and that I was on my own. Sue could not feed, bathe, or dress herself without assistance however, the type of assistance she needed was not medical personnel. This became the defining moment of what she was classified as, a person treated under Custodial Care.

CUSTODIAL CARE refers to non-skilled, personal care, such as help with activities of daily living like bathing, dressing, eating, getting in or out of a bed or chair, moving around, and using the bathroom. It may also include care that most people can do themselves, like using eye drops.

https://www.medicare.gov/files/ask-medicare-types-of-care.pdf

Custodial Care is the purgatory of all levels of care, which no one apparently helped with. It was rapidly determined that Insurance (at least my insurance) did not pay for Custodial Care. Starting out in this long drawn out affair, I spoke with the Insurance for the first time, one of many ridiculously and horrifying conversations. I was told they could sell me a Custodial Care policy for Sue.

It would cost approximately two thousand dollars a month, and it would be an eighty percent coverage policy. I discovered that in order to have anything, and everything supply wise for Sue's care it had to be specifically underwritten within the policy or it would automatically be denied. Therefore, leaving even the most rudimentary of items such as adult diapers off the list would be grounds for denial for that item. I ultimately passed on the policy due to the risk of denial for most basic services, not to mention the burden of shelling out two thousand dollars for the prospect of the extra coverage each month.

Sue's health coupled with what was beginning to be amassing medical bills left our situation feeling dire. I was leaving work early, and missing days outright at a job I had to maintain otherwise there would be no Insurance. Every day was beginning to be a struggle, but I tried not to become flustered at what my life was turning into. Even then I fleetingly realized that missing a day of work in the grand scheme of things was ultimately necessary sometimes for the sake of my own sanity.

CHAPTER THREE

The Diagnoses

I was working full time when caregiving started, in fact I did not know I was a caregiver as of yet. The illness was horrific; whatever Sue was suffering from was undeniably terrible. "My back hurts where they did that spinal tap," she cried out several times. We returned to the Neurologist who had conducted the tests to hear the results of a Spinal Tap, and MRI. The doctor informed us he believed he had a conclusive diagnosis.

Finally maybe we can get some treatment and put this behind us, I thought to myself.

I was experiencing severely varying emotions. I was happy that we would finally know what we were dealing with, yet I was in shock at the same time. What exactly was happening, and what would happen?

"I'm sorry to inform you but I have bad news. It appears you have Multiple Sclerosis (MS) and there is no cure. Now there are drugs that we can give you that will buy you more time and delay the onslaught of the illness." The doctor explained to us.

I suffer from somewhat extensive hearing damage due to a misspent youth. At that moment I didn't know if it was my hearing or if it was the numbness I was feeling that caused the doctor to trail off. I regained my composure after a minute and attempted to continue listening. The doctor informed us based on the results of the tests, as well as the appearance of lesions on her brain meant she without a doubt had MS. The doctor informed me that Sue's lesions were an exact copy of one another. After we left the doctor's office and returned home I immediately began to scour the internet to learn more about the disease. The Google searches were providing relieve and terror simultaneously. I needed someone to rush into the house and disconnect the internet to save me from my agonizing and never ending searches. Generally speaking or at least based on my extensive internet searching I immediately began to wonder if Sue was misdiagnosed due to information indicating lesions in MS patients are different sizes and not the exact same copy of each other. I contemplated this possibility for some time but ultimately knew whatever the doctors had planned would be her best hope. Sue was prescribed the drug Copaxone, which was administered via injection.

COPAXONE® (glatiramer acetate injection) is indicated for the treatment of patients with relapsing forms of multiple sclerosis. www.copaxone.com

We obtained an auto injector which required loading the needle into the tube before injecting it into her body. Due to the burns Sue obtained from the 1981 car wreck she was left with very limited injection sites. Sue quickly tired of the injections and desired to quit the medicine. She felt as though it was not helping her condition. "I want to stop this treatment, I do not like it and it is not helping me anymore," Sue complained.

Each time we attempted to stop Copaxone her entire body essentially began a meltdown. Her muscles became like jelly forcing us to continue the shots. I called and spoke with the drug maker after experiencing this.

"Why can't I take her off the drug without having this type of side effect?" I asked.

"We have never had this problem before we will have to look into what you're saying." A representative said.

With several unsuccessful attempts to remove her from the drug we continued injecting Copaxone. I felt at this time as if I was prepared for what was coming. I researched MS thoroughly and I knew what to expect, at least I thought I knew. It wasn't until later that we realized how far in decline she actually was. It was not until later that the reason for the failed attempts at taking her off the Copaxone was revealed, she was slowly starving to death and no one knew it.

I soon realized how valuable resources were at this point. I contacted the MS Society to determine if I qualified for any type of assistance for Sue. A person from the local chapter of the MS Society arrived to survey Sue. She was able to help paint us a clearer picture of where Sue stood in the process of the disease, and helped us obtain a scooter for Sue.

"Your wife will be in a wheelchair soon." The MS resprenstive said turning towards me as she left.

The scooter quickly became a blessing, giving Sue a sense of new self-freedom. While her mobility had begun to be limited she could now move around in our house without fear of falling as long as someone helped her into and out of the scooter. She operated the scooter amazingly well. The vehicle we owned also was seemingly a blessing.

Months passed before our initial appointment materialized at the University of Texas Southwestern MS clinic in Dallas, Texas. Our Chevrolet HHR provided the room to fold down the scooter into the vehicle without having to purchase an added expense of a wheelchair lift. Once we got into The MS clinic I found it much easier to allow the valet people to park our car and get Sue out of the car at the door of the entrance to the building. Upon our arrival I continually exploited the valet parking service simply for the extra assistance.

The valet parkers were helpful and would do whatever they could to help us in and out of the building. Each time we drove up to the clinic, there they were to help us out. They were truly blessings to us as they moved to help us get out of the car and then go and park our car then bring our car back to us and help us back into the car for only five dollars.

Sue regularly accompanied me to places like Walmart, just to get her out of the house. I was amazed at times that we did not end up on People of Walmart due to our appearance, and the overwhelming confused faces we encountered. Younger children appeared scared as we passed them, and often hid peeking behind their parent's legs. Since Sue could no longer operate the scooter I would press the handle from behind me while pushing the grocery cart ahead of me. At times I literally felt as though I was stretched too thin, and the cart as I loaded it up with food got too heavy to push with one arm. Once the cart was too heavy to push I ultimately was forced to push the cart half way down the aisle, stop and then rush to retrieve Sue. It became unreasonable, and I was unable to do both simultaneously. I had nowhere to turn to, and no one to help me. Jennifer was at school, and Travis was with his children in Missouri. I desperately wanted anybody to appear and say, "Hey let me get this for you." No one did. We were struggling to find what was really wrong with Sue so we could find successful treatments.

Officially I noticed on paper work of the MS clinic that sometimes the paperwork would say MS and sometimes it would say *an unspecified breakdown of the central nervous system*. Therefore I am still not clear in just knowing what illness Sue really had. Life still has some normalcy to it. I could go to work and Sue could take care of herself.

We got the ramp from The Texas Department of Assistive and Rehabilitative Services (DARS).

They came and inspected the ramp. The ramp was twenty feet short. I had companied, "The ramp goes right into the mud." I could not put Sue in the mud and get her to the car. So after

DARS came out and saw what was the problem then they sent workers out to extend the ramp to the driveway and home. Things were changing fast though as we kept on this path that had been given us.

I obtained a mobile chair called The Hover Round from my Insurance Company. It was too big for our little home. It had a joy stick and Sue could not operate the joy stick well. She kept running into walls and objects. I would take Sue outside in the Hover Round. I would walk behind her and move the joy stick for her and take her down the ramp and around the house. We would set under a tree in the yard and talk. She would only take about twenty minutes outside before she wanted to go back into the house. I thought fresh air was good for her. We spent some beautiful moments talking to each other there under the tree. Life was somewhat in decline at this time; although, Sue could still take care of herself. I would run to town real quick to get food and supplies knowing she was good for a little while at home by herself.

Later on I gave the Hover Round to the Methodist man who would come to our home and give us communion. He loaded the chair up into his truck. He told me later, "You will love to know I gave that Hover Round to a man who can now get out of his house and go to the pond and go fishing!"

"Beautiful" I told him. "That is a blessing to hear."

CHAPTER FOUR

New Beginnings

We were doing our best to adjust to our new and unwanted lifestyle. Our daughter Jennifer was at this point in her first few years of college. She had offered to leave school in an attempt to help care for Sue. I fended her off knowing that her full paid scholarship wouldn't wait, and I wanted her to get her education. On weekends she would travel two and a half hours from her campus to spend time with us and work at her local job. One weekend I received a frantic call from her while I was at work.

"Hey dad it's Jennifer."

"Yeah." I stated.

"I'm on my way back to the house. Mom fell and she was having a hard time getting through to me at work because nobody could understand her." Jennifer said.

Oh God, I thought to myself.

It was apparent she could no longer stay home alone, but what was I going to do? I had no resources to help me, and I couldn't possibly afford to hire someone to take care of her while I worked. It was close to the end of my shift and I returned home. Jennifer stayed home and waited for my return, while Sue rested. Jennifer told me about the horror of what had occurred. A coworker of hers had kept hanging up when Sue called thinking she was intoxicated due to her slurring words. It was getting to the point that no one could understand her and Society almost didn't seemed prepared to deal with it.

The only plausible conclusion I could ascertain was to find Sue a Nursing home, or an Assisted Living Center. We found out that we could not go into an Assistive Living Center due to her age. Sue was too young under their policies. At this time we were both in our late forties.

I took Sue to a nursing home following the latest incident. We were disheartened to learn Sue could not be placed into a nursing home due to our income. We grossed more than $2,000 a month between her disability and my income. The Activities Director approached me with other possibilities,

"I think we have another way we can help you." She said.

"Okay, what if any options do we have?" I asked somewhat desperately.

"I'll make a call this afternoon for someone to come out to your house for an evaluation."

"Whatever help we can get, please." I said.

Unbeknownst to me, she had contact a local Hospice Charter. Sue and I had returned to our home, and I was dismayed when the intake worker arrived. He introduced himself and completed the assessment of Sue for the "intake process."

"I thought Hospice was for terminal patients." I stated.

"Hospice is not just for those who are dying. It can be for those with long term illness as well." the man from Hospice explained.

During the "intake process" he explained that Sue was evaluated and would remain in Hospice for approximately six months. At the end of the six month period she would be reevaluated to determine is she was declining, or making progression. If she were progressing she would be removed from the Hospice care at that time.

Sue and I had recently discussed what she wanted. With an incurable disease progressing I needed to know what she wanted.

We discussed Power of Attorneys (PoAs), Do Not Resuscitate (DNR) orders, and the possibility of donating her body upon her death to science for research. I Google Power of Attorney and here is what I found:

"A power of attorney is a legal document that gives someone you choose the power to act in your place. In case you ever become mentally incapacitated, you'll need what are known as "durable" powers of attorney for medical care and finances."

https://www.google.com/#q=powers+of+attorneys+

"Advance directives are legal documents that allow you to convey your decisions about end-of-life care ahead of time. They provide a way for you to communicate your wishes to family, friends and health care professionals, and to avoid confusion later on." He said.

Here is the general information where we pulled our PoAs down from. Just download and go with witness and file away as you need.

Declaration for Mental Health Treatment —This document allows you to make decisions in advance about mental health treatment and specifically three types of mental health treatment: psychoactive medication, convulsive therapy and emergency mental health treatment. The instructions that you include in this declaration will be followed only if a court believes that you are incapacitated to make treatment decisions. Otherwise, you will be considered able to give or withhold consent for the treatments.

Directive to Physicians and Family or Surrogates Form — This form is designed to help you communicate your wishes about medical treatment at some time in the future when you are unable to make your wishes known because of illness or injury.

Medical Power of Attorney Form — Except to the extent you state otherwise, this document gives the person you name as your agent the authority to make any and all health care decisions for you in accordance with your wishes, including your religious and moral beliefs, when you are no longer capable of making them yourself.

Out-of-Hospital Do Not Resuscitate Information & Form (PDF) — This form instructs emergency medical personnel and other health care professionals to forgo resuscitation attempts and to permit the patient to have a natural death with peace and dignity. This order does NOT affect the provision of other emergency care including comfort care.

Statutory Durable Power of Attorney — This form is for designating an agent who is empowered to take certain actions regarding your property. It does not authorize anyone to make medical and other healthcare decisions for you."

https://www.dads.state.tx.us/news_info/publications/handbooks/advancedirectives.html

(Please note I am not a lawyer or CPA, any questions on PoAs or Advance Directives direct to a Lawyer or Certified Public Account.)

When I was in my early thirties my mother was diagnosed with a rare disease known as *Sjogren's Syndrome*, the syndrome is categorized by white blood cells attacking various glands of the body. Even today there is no cure or presentable treatment available. I remember vividly the day she passed away due to complications of the disease. I entered the room and witnessed nurses desperately attempting to remove fluid from her lungs via suction. I slowly walked into the connected bathroom, ignoring the revolting condition it was left in. I dropped to my knees and prayed to God, pleading for her suffering to end. I finally left the bathroom and reentered her room as dawn was approaching along the horizon, a ray of sunshine peeked through the window and shown upon my mother's face as she took her last breath. The doctors approached my father following her death.

"Would you consider donating your wife's body so that we may gain valuable information through research?" The doctor asked.

"No." He replied instantly.

At the time of her death in the 90's, especially in rural Missouri where my family lived it was unheard of to donate a loved one's body. I understood to a point why my father was so adamantly against donation, but I was always bothered by the opportunity that was missed. I imagined the silver lining blessing of her death knowing that someone else one day could have been spared the pain my mom endured. I shared my thoughts on the subject with Sue and we agreed that her death could maybe in turn help others.

"I agree to let John turn my body over to UT Southwestern so my body can be studied," Sue told the intake man.

We discussed at length with the Hospice intake worker what steps needed to be taken to obtain the documents Sue needed, as well as body donation. He directed me to go online to find blank documents that needed to be completed. He additionally informed us that UT Southwestern handled body donation. Before long I had all of the paperwork acquired, and completed. The Power of Attorneys became one of the utmost important documents in our lives.

The following are known as Advance Directives (AD). They are extremely important in care giving so that no one else or group can come into your environment and tell you how you need to care. The only exception to these AD's or PoA's is Abuse and that is not tolerated in caregiving.

(See Our Advance Directives in the back of book in Chapter 19).

I determined after our placement in Hospice, that as a caregiver I could place Sue into Respite Care for a week. I Google Respite Care:

"Respite care is the provision of short-term accommodation in a facility outside the home in which a loved one may be placed. This provides temporary relief to those who are caring for family members, who might otherwise require permanent placement in a facility outside the home."

https://www.google.com/#q=Respite+care

My insurance denied my initial request for Respite Care stating it was not covered. I fervently tried to explain that I needed a break. I needed a few days to myself to recover and reboot from the insurmountable stress I felt every day. After losing yet another battle in the war between the Insurance and myself I was finally informed that Hospice would cover the stay that I requested. I took Sue to a local nursing home for the first time for what was supposed to be a full week. I found during that week that I spent more time with her there at the nursing home than I did in my home, completely negating the entire purpose of her stay. She called the house on what would end up being her last day in the facility after our conversation.

"They were feeding breakfast this morning and they ran out of food." She said.

"What do you mean they ran out of food?" I asked.

"They ran out of food and there's nothing for me to eat now, and some old man keeps following me around."

After all was said and done my experience with this first Hospice was one of sheer disappointment. They were a startup that left me with a bad taste in my mouth. After the debacle of what was supposedly her care I immediately removed her from the nursing home facility. Despite some of my feelings there were some positives that came from this Hospice organization. Many of the staff made up for our feelings of discontent. We had a wonderful bath lady who would come and shower Sue in the shower as well as fantastic LVN's, RN's and an amazing Chaplain.

One afternoon the Chaplin arrived from Hospice to visit with us. When he arrived I was in the middle of a conversation with a representative with my Insurance Company who told me that the Insurance was not covering the Hospice cost.

"Hey do you know that you guys are not getting paid because the paperwork was not filed out correctly with the Insurance Company?" I asked the Chaplain after hanging up the phone.

"Oh really?" He replied.

That was the last I saw of that Hospice group. I had only a fifteen thousand dollar life time benefit with my Insurance Company for Hospice care. The Hospice later refilled the claim that was denied, and was paid all of the fifteen thousand dollars. That was my lifetime benefit with my Insurance Company, leaving me with nothing to fall back on. With Sue leaving Hospice I had to make some more changes. I needed to find help and find it quickly. It was necessary to find a person who would come into my home and take care of my wife so I could continue to work full time.

We soon decided to seek the advice of a lawyer in Dallas named Jean DeWald. It became apparent that Sue would soon not be able to make rational decisions. We need to protect ourselves and each other. I needed to extend Sue's wishes to legal binding court documents to protect us, and make sure they were probably abided by. Our lawyer turned out to be rich blessings for us. She was immensely helpful in more areas then I could have ever dreamed of.

In addition to the Power of Attorneys, we had obtained, Jean helped us to draw up a Will for our lives. We did a Will for Sue and a Will for me. Based on our conversations I began keeping a journal to help protect myself. I could never have imagined how important the PoA's and journal together became to us. It made all the difference from the start to the end of caregiving. The journal allotted me the ability to track everything related to Sue's care including her medications, the side effects, bathing times, allergies, and a variety of other components. The paperwork helped to facilitate everything that needed to be done. We had our Will's finalized and filed away beside the PoA's. When we needed the PoA, all we had to do was to pull them out in emergencies. Any trip to a doctor or hospital meant the PoA was pulled out of my files and taken with us.

I called Attorney Jean DeWald and told her Sue and I needed to file Chapter 7 Bankruptcy. The cost of Sue's care was starting to become insurmountable, and I needed some financial security. Not to mention I knew any of Sue's debt would still linger upon her death. I would literally be living one paycheck away from homelessness every month. We set an appointment with Jean and arrived with all of our bills to be examined.

The lawyer commented that we were better prepared than most people who came into her office. The laws for bankruptcy had changed and required those who filed to complete financial courses online. Sue's health made it difficult motor skill wise for her to navigate through websites. I made Sue sit at the computer and I would click the mouse for her while she watched the bankruptcy videos.

"This is dumb," said Sue.

"I agree but we have to do it," I replied.

In 2010 we were required to attend a creditors meeting. This meeting was conducted at the Federal Building in Dallas with a Trustee. It provides any creditors the opportunity to challenge including your debt in the filing. The Trustee also has the opportunity to review all of the paperwork and ask questions in regards to our filing. We arrived at the meeting and once our names were called Sue wheeled her scooter up to the table, and I sat down with Jean, and the Trustee.

"What's wrong with your wife?" The Trustee asked.

"Honestly we don't know. She has a diagnosis but it's still kind of up in the air." I replied.

The Trustee told our lawyer something causing Jean to quickly grab her note book and scribble away. Sue had several "not at fault" car accidents that were still in the civil process. The Trustee gave us any settlements that may come from the car accidents. Any money collected on the accidents was to be given to us and not to our creditors. I took all of our unsecured debt and walked away from them in Chapter 7 Bankruptcy. I freed up enough money to help continue the care of Sue which was my top priority.

The process of finding a worker had begun; I now had control of my finances and could hire someone to care for Sue during the day. It was essential to take off work to find a worker and then take another week to ten days to train that person before I could go back to work. I called our previous Hospice group and asked for a "setter list." A setter list contained people who volunteered at residences of people attended to by Hospice and sat with them. I called everyone on the list, searching for anyone interested in employment as a sitter. In turn those I contacted who were not interested help spread the word I was looking for an employee. I kept my home open for a week in order to conduct interviews on anyone that applied. Before long the list of people I interviewed included Hospice workers, and others. It took a week to process all of the paperwork and to hire a person. I made sure to include Sue's input for which she preferred to have with her during the day while I was gone. My expectations of my newly hired employee consisted of tending to Sue's needs such as administrating medication, feeding, showering, and using the bathroom.

The business was the business of taking care of my wife. Based on Sue's input we hired a young single mother on March 3, 2010. Prior to hiring her however, I in essence had a meltdown. I had an epiphany that I would be doomed should something happen to her while she was on the "job."

How do I protect myself, I wondered?

I began looking into the issue and speaking with different Attorneys. It was suggested that I call a Certified Public Accountant (CPA). I called the first CPA I found in the phonebook.

"Can you help me set up a business in my home to help me take care of my wife so I can work?" I asked.

"Well yes we can do that for $20." She replied.

That is exactly what I need, I thought to myself.

I called and spoke with the Internal Revenue Service (IRS) as well to get any and all information I could. Upon speaking with the IRS they informed me of potential fines I could face if the business was not executed properly.

Oh my God how can I run this business? I thought to myself.

What first seemed to be a simple task quickly spiraled out of control as I obsessively contacted everyone I could think of to try and protect myself? I called and spoke with my home insurance provider. I told my Agent that I was setting up a business in my home so my wife could be cared for better when I was not there.

"You are paying this person a salary?" He asked.

"Yes of course. Will my home insurance cover her if she got hurt?" I asked.

"No it will not cover an employee. You will need a workman's comp package to do that."

"What would a workman's comp package come to?" I asked.

"Approximately $2000 a month,"

"Oh my God I cannot afford that." I said.

"Let me call the Home Office and see what we can do." He replied.

A few days later the home insurance Agent called.

"We found you a $500,000 workman's comp package for $350 a year." He said.

"Great have them send me the policy then please." I said.

I decided to take this employee to I-Hop for a business dinner so that we could discuss what wheels were set in motion. I drew up a contract and had the term "being there" placed explicitly within the contract. Her interpretation of "being there" unfolded to be quite different than mine. My thought was to "being there" in the room and help Sue with her needs. She evidently thought the term "being there" meant she could talk on her phone constantly, and fill up my DVR with Lifetime Network movies as long as she was there. Sue's feelings towards her became quite clear, and I got the distinct impression she was starting to act out. Sue's way of acting out consisted of echoing a constant whine, and making sometimes outlandish demands. As her disease progressed Sue became demanding, but I couldn't blame her. It was the last bit of control she still obtained in her world, which seemed to be shrinking by the day as she declined. Sue demanded a Chap Stick in one hand, Kleenex's at her will, and a computer game uploaded from Facebook. She knew she was obviously not receiving the care or companionship she desired.

I still felt as though I was working a full time job at home and at work. I would come home to more of a mess then I was use to and suddenly taking care of Sue on top of household chores felt overbearing. One evening I was in disarray. I looked everywhere for my pajamas and could absolutely not find my pajamas anywhere. I turned to Sue and she sat pecking away at her computer nonstop laughing. As her speaking became more difficult we started to rely on communication through her typing on the computer.

"What's so funny?" I asked somewhat irritably.

"God hid your pajamas." She typed out.

Sue's grasp on reality was somewhat beginning to slip. Something I myself chose to attribute to the lesions and spots on her brain. She was beginning to become confused in certain aspects and was unaware of what was occurring in the world and more importantly around her.

I used a new and somewhat unconventional way to communicate with the caretaker I had hired. I used a book on the table to leave instructions on what Sue needed for the day. The employee could also leave notes but more importantly was required to log medications, showers, and various hygienic matters. The employee took notes in the book of calls I missed and made appointments for Sue and I. I made it known in the beginning that Sue needed to be allowed the opportunity to complete whatever she felt able to do. She was declining and every day seemed to bring the fear that more and more was slipping away from her.

In a sense she was still somewhat mobile as she could maneuver about our seemingly small mobile home. During the day she would sit at her computer on Facebook, or emailing family. Sue's entire family resided in the Midwest, mainly Missouri. We had relocated to Texas in the late 90's so that I could work on a Master's degree. After we moved we still made trips to Missouri to see mainly her family, but after she fell ill it was almost impossible to even attempt the eight hour drive. I knew Sue desperately missed her family but the only connection she could make with them was through the internet.

In May of 2010 Jennifer graduated from college, and we were unable to attend. I was out of time with work having missed so many days all stemming from the care of Sue. Luckily our care taker was able to access the live stream of the graduation and play it for Sue. I know she sat at the computer with tears in her eyes. It was a proud moment for the both of us and I was grateful she was at least able to watch it. Jennifer returned from college and began living at our home again. She was having direct interaction with the caretaker and helping out as she could while she worked full time at a local grocery chain called H-E-B.

One day Jennifer called me to warn me of something sinister.

"I just thought I should warn you, mom put a hit out on you." She said slowly.

"What? What?" I asked.

Jennifer relayed the message directly from Sue's Facebook page.

"My husband works at…..I wished someone would go up there and kill him." The message stated.

Wow…the spots on her brain has got to be responsible for this, I thought to myself.

Jennifer knew Sue generally used the same password for a majority of websites and or accounts. She was able to essentially "hack" into her account and remove the content. Sue had a fascination with the games available on Facebook. She regularly played games sometimes for hours on end. But of course what else was there readily available for her to do? While playing these games she regularly added people or persons she was unfamiliar with as friends. This made me nervous to say the least.

For months when I came out of work I would do a one hundred and eighty degree look around. I would watch my back as I drove to the house trying to see if I could find someone following me. This led me to seek out guidance from others who maybe felt the same suffering I did. I started to go to a support group at the local Hospital. Sue was not bad yet and most people in the group were not where I was at or where I was going. Most were dealing with Alzheimer's and I was dealing with the breakdown of the Central Nervous System. I went for a couple of months then I left the group. There were more troubles to come in caregiving in this family. Sue's spots on her brain were increasingly affecting her decision making.

Up to this point I thought life had been rough, but it got even rougher than anything I could have ever expected. Yet again I was wrong, I didn't know what was in store for us and I wished somebody could have given me a heads up. Challenges came in many forms. One such challenge was voting.

It was election time. Sue wanted to go vote. During election time Sue and I would head to our local polling place. The first time we attempted to vote I realized how hard something easy as voting that minute could become a challenge. I noticed The Electioneer glance from my peripheral vision while I was tending to Sue's needs. I told the Electioneer,

"She is going to need my assistance casting her ballot, and I was not sure of the process of how we do that?"

The Electioneer Officer and I spoke for a few moments and the Electioneer asked me,

"Raise your right hand and repeat after me,"

"Do you swear that you will just help her and not vote for her?"

"I do," I replied.

I did not know it was possible to be sworn in to assist in her with voting. I would roll Sue over to the voting booth and I would let her read the page and I would ask her 1, 2, or 3? She would give me one finger up, two fingers up and three fingers up to tell me which one to vote then I pressed the button on the number of fingers she showed me. We voted at least three times like this. It gave Sue value as a person to be able to vote.

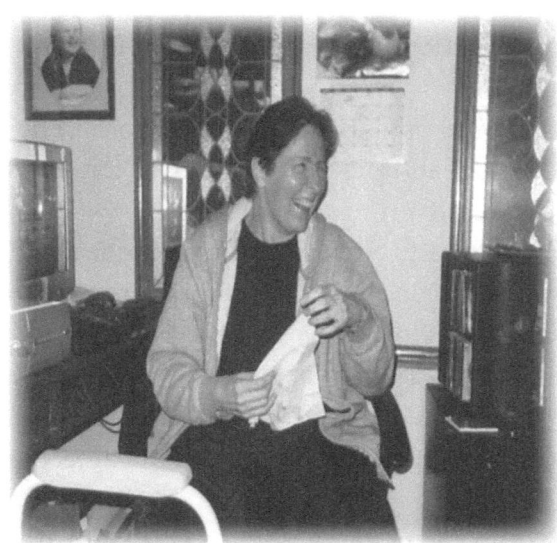

CHAPTER FIVE

Life Has Changed

One day I took Sue to the MS clinic, and after our visit we waited for valet to bring the car to us. By this time, Sue had lost the motor function ability to press the forward and reverse handles all together. I would walk in front of the scooter all the time and push the handle forward for her. Sometimes I think Sue would crank the speed up and run me over for fun. After hitting me Sue's face would immediately light up with a mischievous grin, as she attempted to not burst into uncontrollable laughter. Something she was widely known for, sometimes even in the most unconventional places.

I am not exactly sure how it happened but, as the car pulled up and I hit the handle to bring Sue towards the car we hit a curb in the process. Sue went flying out of the scooter, taking a tumble for the worse. The expressions on the valet's faces were enough to make me want to crawl into a hole from embarrassment and sorrow. That day hurt both of us. Even when going through the everyday motions left me feeling open, and exposed. The opportunity was always present for any type of accident to occur at any time. I felt the urge to guard Sue, but it was impossible. I could not protect her from anything, especially the damager her own body was doing to itself.

I took Sue back to the Urologist once her ability to speak began to dissipate. When we were out of the house our ability to communicate was hindered without her computer. I decided to buy her a small lap top so she could type what she needed to say. Sue could still speak, but her slurred speech made it daunting for others to understand. She relied on using the computer to get her message across for fear of miscommunication. While in the office she started pecking away on her computer. She motioned for me to show her computer to the doctor. I pulled the laptop and swiveled it around to show the doctor without looking at what she had typed. I looked below just as the doctor did to see the message.

He is mean, he is mean, he is mean, is what she wrote on the laptop.

I looked at the Doctor and immediately told him about her spots on the brain. The Doctor informed me he was required by law to report the incident to Adult Protective Services (APS). I came home a few days later and an investigator was sitting with Sue at her computer.

"Go back outside and stay out there until I call you back in," the APS office said.

So I went outside and realized just how beautiful a day it was. I sat down in a lawn chair and appreciated the things around me that I hadn't really seen lately. I basked in the sunlight and relaxed, while listening to the birds singing. I had my one and only real break for the first time since 2007, and it was wonderful. The thirty minutes did not last nearly long enough before the APS officer called me back into the house.

"Thank you." I said.

"For what?" She replied.

"For that blessed, peaceful break you just gave me."

There was nothing I could do in this situation. How could I possibly defend myself against this kind of accusation? Sue and I had our problems in the past, but I was doing the best I could for her with the limited resources I had at my disposal. I answered her questions and she left shortly thereafter. Before leaving she handed me her card, several days later I called her,

"Where do we stand here?" I asked.

"There is no Preponderance of Evidence." She replied.

"I love my wife dearly, and I do the best I can for her." I stated.

"I know you do." She replied.

The investigation was over and I felt a sense of relieve. That perhaps the worst was over and we could continue just focusing on Sue's care. This single mother worked for a few more weeks before turning in her two weeks notice. Luckily with Jennifer back at the house we delayed the search for a new caregiver to sit with Sue while I was at work.

I didn't expect to be so worn out as a caregiver. I was so tired, weak, and far out of my comfort zone, I was beyond overwhelmed. Each day I would get up and hit the floor running. Sue would get me up at all hours of the night. Sometimes it was something she really needed, most time it was for a Kleenex or Chap Stick. Caregiving had become physically and emotionally draining. I knew that this caregiving experience took years off my life and yet still more changes came to us.

Sue soon developed *Dysphagia*. *Dysphagia* in lameness terms was swallowing difficulties. In conjunction with her difficulty speaking Sue was also having difficulty eating. Every day varied in what she could and could not eat. What was easy for her to eat one day was impossible the next day. One evening I cooked dinner and was putting away dishes while she ate when I heard the very distinctive sound of her chocking. I rushed over to her and performed the Heimlich Maneuver on her by getting behind her and pushing upward into her stomach to force the food out of her throat. Over the course of her illness, I was forced to perform the Heimlich Maneuver three times. There was no time to think, only time for me to react. I would feed her the way I knew she could eat, making cooking very tricky.

Meal-On-Wheels started to deliver to the house for a period of time, bringing her lunch during the day. Years ago prior to Sue becoming sick she had volunteered with the organization, and had herself delivered meals to members of the community. I felt a twinge of uneasiness; I never could have imagined we would end up using their services. The irony did not sit well with me at all. It was good to know that while I was away there was a meal for her ready to go. Over time though they became useless as her difficulty swallowing progressed.

In the last few days I remember Sue having her voice we had a short but wonderful conversation.

"Sue will you teach me how to cook?" I asked.

"Yes I will help you cook John," she said to me.

Between my hearing and her speech we were made *The Odd Couple* at best. I searched the cabinets and located her old recipe box. It was a dark green color Tupperware box with plenty of varying recipes in it. Between Sue's help and the recipe book I felt like I was finally able to hold on to at least one part of our normal life, and that was Sue's cooking.

In June of 2010 I looked down at Sue one day with an epiphany. She was still attempting to eat and eating while one of the most natural things it had become an unrelenting task for us, especially her. While looking at her I realized something was drastically wrong. She looked mere skin and bones and looked as though she was withering away in front of me. I called a local surgeon's office immediately.

I told a staff member of the surgeon's office that I believed my wife was starving. I was given an appointment for the following day for a consultation. I told Sue she was having *nothing by mouth* after midnight, (NPO), to prepare for the consultation. The next day at the surgeon's office I told the nurse, "My wife is starving."

We sat down in the doctor's office, I pointed at Sue, and I explained to Dr. John Sullivan,

"I feared that she is starving to death."

"I have been NPO since midnight," she told Dr. Sullivan.

The doctor asked us to wait there in the room, he left the room, and then when he returned, he requested that we do the labs there in the clinic and then he had us meet him at the Surgery Center an hour later. Sue had a Gastric Feeding Tube, (G-Tube) place in her stomach wall.

"What do we do now?" I asked Dr. Sullivan,

"You will have to give her Jeivty 1.2 nutritional shakes," He answered as he gave me and script for Jevity.

I went to Ennis Medical Supply of Ennis TX. I showed them my Insurance information. The worker informed us that the Insurance had denied coverage for the Jeivty. She informed me that the cost of Jeivty is one dollar and ninety nine cents per can. The doctor ordered Sue to receive one to two cans a day, three times a day. I wondered to myself, *Oh my God what do I do now?* My wife has a feeding tube, the Insurance is refusing to help, and she is looking at this time as if she could die at any moment due to starvation.

So I did what I had to do since the Insurance was refusing to help me. I went to Walgreen's Pharmacy in Ennis, TX to get nutritional supplements. There I bought one month's supply worth of Walgreen nutritional supplements. I bought five cans times thirty days which came to one hundred and fifty cans of supplements a month that Sue needed. The month's price came to two hundred ninety eight dollars and fifty cents per each month. I spoke with the manager of the facility, and requested that she should order more so that Walgreen's would be able to meet our needs. I bought this monthly supply for the months of June, July and August 2010. I had to learn how to feed Sue with a feeding tube.

The feeding tube was something new for us. I had never been in this type of situation and was completely unprepared for dealing with a feeding tube. I had no earthly idea what to possibly do next. He gave me a prescription for Jeivty, a nutritional supplement and told me to go to a medical supply store. He explained the proper way to feed Sue, as well as clean the *stoma* area: where the tube went into her stomach wall. I had purchased a food processor. I thought that perhaps I could process healthy and nutritional food and feed her the processed food through the G-Tube. It is still a new food processor. I quickly came to realize that even the processed food was too thick to make its way through the G-Tube. I was to say the least floored. I had no idea what to possibly do. I was out of options, and was forced to go to Walgreens and purchase their nutritional shakes. For three months I paid around three hundred dollars just to feed Sue through the G-Tube.

In September of 2010 I took Sue to the hospital in town. She was complaining of pain and I knew it was not the type of pain she was use to regularly dealing with. They admitted her due to an inflamed *Pancreas*. A Nutritionist came into our room in the hospital to talk to us about the shakes. She reiterated that Sue needed to be receiving Jeivty 1.2 nutritional shakes. The situation left me feeling embarrassed, and angry. I felt as though I was being scolded and ridiculed, yet no one was offering me assistance to get what I needed. It was as if I was playing a game, and no one had bothered to tell me the rules. Shortly thereafter the hospital visit the Insurance Company agreed to start paying for the Jeivty. I couldn't help but wonder why had they not paid at the beginning of the G-Tube feeding process?

We always had a way for Sue to communicate. Once she lost her ability to speak we would talk to each other using the computer. No matter where we went we would take the mini laptop that I had purchased. One problem with our system was that I constantly lost that darn laptop. Twenty miles down the road after an afternoon trip to the grocery store I remembered that I left the lap top in the Family Bathroom of the store. If one of us needed to use the bathroom it was our best bet of not being stared at or silently ridiculed. We had started to go into the men's bathroom and one time I realized after looking at Sue's face bursting out in laughter when I said out loud, "My God look at all the stalls," not realizing that I was in the women's bathroom. I had quickly come to realize that people were not understanding of our situation unless they had experienced a disabled love one themselves. I immediately turned around and rushed back to the store. I ran to the back of the store where the family bathrooms were located. To my dismay the laptop was not there.

"Shoot!!!" I cried out. "I cannot afford to buy another one."

That laptop was the center of communication for Sue, especially while out of the house. I walked to the service desk and explained my situation in hopes that somehow it was still there.

"Did somebody turn in a mini laptop by chance?" I asked.

"Hang on." The customer service assistant walked to the back and fumbled around for a minute before returning to the front desk.

"Someone brought it up here from the back bathroom." She said.

"Oh thank God!!" I cried out.

I worked my way back to the car with a smile on my face. I was grateful we weren't facing another additional expenditure. Sue smiled too when she saw I had the laptop in hand. "Thank you," she typed out to me.

I had developed a terrible habit when putting Sue into the car. I would have the laptop in my hand and I would place it on the roof of the car while I transported her from the scooter to the car seat. I would then work my way to the back of our vehicle where I would fold the scooter into the backseat and jump in the car myself. Unfortunately, I would forget to go back for the laptop and it would remain sitting on top the roof of the car until I sat back into the car. Sue would usually whine and push her head upward in an effort to remind me of my mistake. It would usually take a second before I'd realize what I had done and hastily exit the car to grab the laptop.

One day not only did I forget but Sue also forgot about the laptop. I took off from the house with Sue doing fifty miles per hour down the south bound service road. Suddenly I heard something that sounded as though it was flying off the roof of our car.

"What was that?" I asked looking over at Sue.

Suddenly Sue glanced at me with wide eyes and I immediately knew.

"That was the laptop wasn't it?" I asked.

Sue immediately pursed her lips and violently shook her head up and down.

After our appointment I took Sue home and went looking for the laptop. I found it lying in pieces across the service road. We went for weeks without the laptop that we desperately needed. I borrowed a larger laptop from a coworker but it was way too big for Sue's needs. I applied for a credit card and luckily was approved so I took Sue to Best Buy and bought her another laptop with insurance covering it. Sue later spilt a drink across the keyboard causing it to no longer work; thankfully with a little hindsight we were covered. I went back to Best Buy with my insurance paperwork for the computer and got my money back and went back to Walmart and found an identical copy of our original laptop that flew off the roof of the car. We were back in business again.

CHAPTER SIX

Learning how Insurance works

In August, 2010 I got very hungry. I have a monthly food budget of three hundred dollars for food. Sue's nutritional drinks from Walgreens were around three hundred dollars a month. Therefore, I called my Insurance Company in Dallas, Texas. I spoke with a Customer Advocate.

"We need to compare apples to oranges," I said to them on the phone.

"If I took my wife to a hospital, would the Insurance cover their part, correct?" I asked.

"Yes." The representative responded.

The representative proceeded to explain the in network policy.

"If I needed a wheel chair, you would not pay for it?" I asked.

"No that is considered Custodial Care, which is not covered by your policy." She responded.

"What about the G-tube that we surgically placed within my wife, you paid for that?" I asked.

"Yes we did." She said.

"Well then explain to me why in the world would you not pay for the nutritional drinks that go into the G-tube, which she requires to be kept alive with?" I asked.

"Hang on," she said while placing me on hold.

"Yes we will pay for the nutritional drinks." She said.

"Good then please send me some claim forms for me to fill out, because I have medical supplements for this G-tube that needs to be paid for." I replied to her.

My Insurance Company sent the claim forms, I gathered my claim information, and then I returned them in the mail to the Dallas office.

I contacted the Dallas office at a later date to inquire as to why my claims had still not been covered. They informed me that I needed a *letter from the doctor* that stated that Sue required the nutritional drinks. So I contacted Dr. Sullivan and requested the letter. I waited, waited and waited. I finally contacted Dr. Sullivan again and requested for a copy of the entire medical file of the G-Tube placement procedure. His office supplied this information to me, at the personal cost of fifty dollars and forty two cents. I made a copy for myself. Then I copied and sent the entire file which included the *doctors' letter* to the Dallas office for my Insurance Company.

I waited some more and then contacted the Dallas office yet again, I inquired what was the hold up on the situation now? The Customer Advocate informed me that something was wrong with the letter. That the letter did not fully explain why she needed what was being asked for. The run around puzzled me.

"Do you have the copy that I sent you, the medical file I mean?" I asked.

"Yes we do." She stated.

I gathered my copy of the information that I sent to them, then I read my copy of the letter to the Customer Advocate to ascertain what else I would possibly need. I read this, letter from the doctor back to her.

"Well I believe we do have everything we need." She said.

After months of haggling my Insurance Company sent the check to cover the cost of the Walgreen's shakes I was forced to purchase. My initial reaction was one of delight; I had finally won a battle against Goliath. For the millionth time I was wrong, again. The amount of the check barely covered a two week supply that I was out of pocket for. My original claim of nine hundred dollars was for three months' worth of nutritional shakes. I got a check for one hundred dollars and twenty eight cents. I called my Insurance Company up being angrier than ever before.

"That's all we are going to pay." The Insurance Representative said to me.

"We will see." I replied.

This conversation set me on a collision course for an asinine and ridiculous fight with my Insurance Provider. The fight over nutritional shakes to keep Sue alive lasted over many months. I would use a land line phone whenever calling my Insurance Company. As soon as I would put my insurance identification number into the Dallas office system I would automatically be placed on hold, a hold that lasted for hours. I did not have the time to stay hanging onto a phone; I needed to care for my wife. The office started doing things that were utterly mind boggling. They would send me confusing letters attempting to throw me off course. They wanted a *provider and date of service*, which was impossible to provide since I bought an over the counter supplement. It was *medically necessary* for Sue to have those shakes in order to survive, but I somehow could not prove it.

They stone walled my claim and it became very apparent they were not going to pay. One evening I had an especially difficult care giving night. I did my daily calling to my Insurance Company. I called after 7 P.M. which is when apparently the Dallas office closes and the customer service calls are rerouted to Albuquerque, New Mexico. I called them and was doing my usually complaining of why they were not paying for a *medical necessary* item for life. The Customer Advocate in Albuquerque started apologizing to me. For two hours he told me how sorry he was that the Insurance

Company was treating us like that. He was right, and it suddenly dawned on me how terribly mistreated our situation was.

The Customer Advocate told me to start asking for *reference numbers*. When you call up Insurance Company, if you ask for a reference number they have to keep the conversation. Based on our conversation I called the Dallas office the following evening.

"Are you guys going to pay for a wheelchair?" I asked.

"No. That's a Custodial Care item." The female Dallas Customer Advocate responded.

"Ok. I'd like the reference number for this please." I stated.

That same evening I called the Albuquerque office and gave them the reference number regarding my Dallas conversation.

"Wow that pretty cut and dry." The Albuquerque representative said.

"That's how they are treating my wife and I." I replied.

I had my Insurance Company in two different offices and in two different States saying opposite things. Dallas was treating me terrible, but Albuquerque treated me like a person.

Needless to say I was steaming mad with my Insurance Company for not paying for *medical necessary* items for life. One afternoon in the fall of 2011, I was driving into town when I saw the local district office of Honorable Joe Barton, my US House of Representatives', Representative. I stopped in Joe Barton's office in my Correctional Officer uniform and I began to tell my story to the woman behind the desk.

"No do not tell me, you will just have to tell your story again. You need to talk to Judy." She said.

She disappeared for a few minutes, before returning to the front.

"Come here I have Judy on the line for you." She said.

She lead me into the back room. I saw a big, beautiful couch and a huge oak wood coffee table with a phone off the hook lying upon the table. Elections were coming and I was hopeful I might obtain some type of help. I began with telling Judy of my problem with my Insurance Company not paying for *medical necessary* nutritional drinks and how it had taken a toll on my wife and I.

"What do you want us to do about it?" She asked.

"Oh you just did not say that to me. I want you to know ma'am I am a staunch Republican. I go into the ballet box a lot and hit straight party ticket. Do you hear how mad I am? I am standing in your office in this city, and if you let me walk out of your office this mad, I will walk into the ballot box in November and vote straight Democrat party ticket." I explain to her.

"We can do an insurance inquiry." She replied immediately.

"That's a start." I said.

The paperwork was filled out and sent to an office in Arlington, Texas.

(See First letter I sent to the Honorable Congressmen Joe Barton in the back of the book in Chapter 19.)

CHAPTER SEVEN

Crazy Days

October 25, 2010 started out to be a beautiful day; however, weather reports indicated that severe weather could strike our area. Suddenly I heard my NOAA weather radio alarm begin to blare, snapping me from my mundane daily care giving routine. The weather radio blasted the report across the speakers with the distinctive alarms deafening through the silent house.

"Navarro County is now under a Tornado Warning. Anyone in the area needs to take cover immediately. The Tornado is currently in Emhouse, and could possibly affect Rice, Alma, Ellis County, and Kaufman Counties."

"We got to get to the High School Sue that Tornado is only nine miles away from us." I shouted to Sue.

The High School was approximately one mile South of us, and was our town's designated evacuation point for Tornado's. Sue was wearing only a T-Shirt, diaper and socks, forcing me to dress her rather hastily. On a normal day once she was dressed the process of getting Sue out of the house and into the car on average took somewhere between fifteen to twenty minutes. The process included getting the scooter, lifting Sue from the bed to the scooter, dressing her in pants and top, putting her shoes on her feet and lacing her shoes, before heading out the back door down the ramp to the car. After loading Sue into the scooter I opened the back door, revealing hail the size of baseballs. I shut the door and escorted Sue along with the weather radio to our bedroom. I swiftly plugged the weather radio into an outlet having neglected purchasing batteries.

I laid Sue on the floor and put a couple of blankets over her. I went to the front door and looked to my left; the skyline produced a deceiving picture. The sky appeared to literally be severed into two pieces. To my left was a beautiful and serene landscape while a Tornado was descending from the heavens to my right. A loud boom emitted from the sky sending a shockwave through me, as I heard the sound of a freight train barreling towards me. I locked the front door later only wondering what I thought that could have possibly prevented. I ran back to Sue in the bedroom, and began piling every pillow and blanket I could find to put over her.

I lay down next to Sue, and hugged her as tightly as I could through the layer of bedding. The power abruptly ceased to work, taking with it the weather radio lifeline. The house was pierced by the harrowing sound of silence.

"Honey we are going to go to Heaven together!" I yelled.

I quickly said a prayer asking for the Lord to protect us. The lights flickered on and the weather radio returned saying the Tornado was North of us in a neighboring small town. I picked myself off the floor and headed to the front door. I looked to the sky and witnessed two separated pieces of sky abruptly switch places. To the right of me was clear and serene, and the left contained the Tornado which dissipated into the atmosphere.

"Let's get out of here there might be more." I yelled running back to Sue.

I loaded her into the car and we headed to the High School. I rushed Sue to the bathroom in the school and told her I would be right back. I went to the side of the High School and looked out the glass windows.

Oh my God. I blurted to myself.

The school system had just built a brand new Middle school next to the High school, which had not yet opened. Less than a quarter a mile ahead of me laid debris from the school. It was apparent that when the Tornado turned away from our house it struck the school.

"We got to get out of here we are on ground zero where that Tornado touched down." I said after immediately returning to Sue.

I loaded Sue back into the car and followed a Texas State Trooper out of the parking lot. It appeared as if he was surveying the damage to the school. I followed the trooper past the back road of the Middle school. The back wall of the school had dissipated into rubble. I followed the road to the service road running parallel to the interstate in an attempt to complete the five mile loop back to our house. I peered out the driver's side window as countless agencies descended from the highway to the school. Police from neighboring towns, State Troopers, Constables, Rangers, Fire Trucks and Ambulances approached quickly to bring aid to any injured.

The entrance and exit ramps from the highway were blocked preventing anyone from entering or exiting the newly congested area. Traffic clearly slowed to a standstill. Traffic on both side of the interstate and service road were crammed with vehicles. Finally after forty minutes, I got a chance to head North on the service road. I abruptly slammed my breaks on and came to a stop. There was a huge wall cloud one hundred to two hundred feet up in the air and it was turning around and around rather quickly. I heard a car horn blow behind me. I looked back to the truck behind me and pointed up to the turning wall cloud. I thought we were blessed that it did not touch down on top of us as we remained trapped in the one spot. It took an hour to travel what should have been six minutes back to our house. I unloaded Sue and put her back into her hospital bed. I walked outside and began to survey our own damage.

Hail damage struck both our home and the car littering the area with bumps and dents. I was never more grateful to have insurance coverage then I was in that moment.

I was setting in my shift turn out room when I returned to work several days after the unwanted excitement from the tornado, when a Human Resources worker called me to go to the office. She handed me an application for financial help. I thanked her, filled it out, and took it back to the office. A few days later on my day off I received a call from the Warden's Secretary.

"The Warden would like to talk to you today can you come around 2 P.M.?" The warden's secretary asked.

"Well I would say yes but I'm taking care of my wife right now. Is it alright if I bring her to the unit with me?" I replied.

"That would be fine if you brought her." She said.

I dressed Sue and took her with me to the unit. We entered the unit and headed for the office where both the Warden and Assistant Warden were waiting. They had two seats there for us to set in. I moved one of the seats out of the way and gently guided the scooter into the spot where the seat was originally placed before sitting next to Sue.

"Well I did not know why we would be supporting you, but now I see why." The Warden stated.

She walked over and hugged Sue.

"Here is my email address you email me if he does not treat you right." She said.

"I will let you know if John does not treat me right Warden," Sue typing out on her computer.

They gave us a check for around five hundred dollars. I took that email address of the Warden and I emailed her asking, *how may I pray for you?* From time to time she would respond and I would send back a prayer like I do through the Guidepost ministry. That meeting provided more than just financial assistance. There is a lot of stress in working in a prison setting. You obtain stress from every possible direction. The added stress from work suddenly halted. From the Warden all the way down to the Correctional Officers, no one bothered me. Some would listen to me vent, and some would simply pray for me. They provided encouragement that was desperately needed on a daily basis. Every year at the unit in May we have a day called The Employee Appreciation Day. There also a time to remember those who have been killed in the line of duty. I was at home and in the morning time I received a call from my Lieutenant.

"Mr. Patterson can you come to the unit this evening and pray for those who have fallen in the line of duty? I am afraid the unit Chaplain cannot come and since you work in the Chapel so much we would like for you to stand in for the Chaplin." My Lieutenant said to me.

"Yes I would do that for you but can I please bring my wife. I cannot leave her alone?"

"Sure you can bring her with you just come to the back gate."

I was glad the Lieutenant said I could bring her through the back gate. That meant I would not be seen bringing Sue down the slab of the unit in a scooter she could not control. By coming through the back gate no offenders would come into contact with us.

We got there early and no problems getting though the back gate after hours. Sue and I went into the Chapel. What was weird about the evening had nothing to do with Sue. It seems that when I went into prayer for those who had lost their lives. I prayed for the families left behind then I prayed for those in the coming months and years in the future who would in fact lose their lives in the line of duty and those who they were going to be leaving behind. The next evening an officer found me on shift and his eyes got big and he said, "Man, wow, that prayer you said last night! Wow!"

After work one afternoon I stopped and grabbed the mail before heading home. There was an application in Sue's name for a credit card. The last thing I knew we needed was a credit card after Chapter 7 Bankruptcy. I turned to Sue with the application in hand.

"Here is one credit card you are not going to get and charge up." I said as I shredded the credit card application. I did not know it, but Sue called the Police.

"My husband just shredded my mail." She had stated to them.

I heard a knock at the door. I opened it to find two Police officers, a male and a female officer. They came into the house.

"Sir did you shred your wife's mail?" The female officer asked.

"Yes I did." I replied.

The female police officer escorted me outside while the male officer remained inside talking to Sue. I could see she was about to arrest me: since she was going for her handcuffs.

"Ma'am I have Power of Attorney on my wife," I stated.

"You do?" She asked.

"Yes I do." I replied.

"Show me the Power of Attorney." She said.

I took the officer back into my house and pulled out the Power of Attorney in the file cabinet that regards to financials. She read it and called out to the other officer.

"Hey partner he has Power of Attorney." She said.

"He does? Let me see it." He replied.

He read over the document and turned to Sue.

"Ma'am he can shred your mail." The male officer said.

It seemed like situations like these were arising. It felt like a mixture of bad luck, and Sue's degenerating illness. The lesions on her brain began to make her loose grasp on reality. As some point during this time Sue was given a cognitive test. The results revealed she had failed basic questions such as "who" the President was, and what year it was. It indicated that Sue was suffering from possible brain degeneration. It was not the last time police would come into our home.

Several weeks later I was attempting to relax with bear feet while sitting in my favorite chair, watching the news. Sue was buzzing around the house in her scooter. Before I could realize what was happening Sue was running over the top of my foot with the scooter. Pain shot into my foot like I had never felt before. I was screaming out in pain and shouting, probably louder then I intended. What do you think Sue did? She called the Police, which typically when Sue would call she would place the phone down after dialing 911. Making no attempt whatsoever to try and explain what the emergency was, at least in her eyes. I looked up still screaming out in pain and saw the Police Officer standing over me. I did not hear him come through my open door of my home. I immediately explained what had transpired and how she accidently ran over my foot hurting it tremendously. The Police Office made sure there was nothing other than that occurring in my home that night before leaving.

I took the phone off Sue's desk, canceling our land line. I made sure that anyone in the house from that day on had access to a cell phone, but Sue had no access to a phone after that date. I was worried one more frivolous call to law enforcement would send me to jail over Sue's abuse of calling 911.

Jennifer up until this point was living at the house and helping take care of Sue as she could couple with working. After several months of job searching she landed employment with the State of Texas as a Parole Officer stationed a little over an hour away. It became apparent that she was no longer going to be able to stay and take care of Sue while I was at work as our work hours were nearly identical.

She received the job offer in November of 2010 a week or two prior to Thanksgiving and informed me that she was expected to start January 2011. This gave me a few months to start the process over with locating a new worker.

Jennifer volunteered to cook "Thanksgiving dinner" while I was at work. I had asked her to make Sue felt included in cooking dinner. It had been several years since we were able to celebrate Thanksgiving on the actual day and not a week before due to my job. Jennifer had promised me she would and stated she would do the best she could. It was the first time Jennifer had cooked this type of meal and I knew she would feel a little unsteady in doing so.

Sue motioned for Jennifer to go to the computer desk. She obliged and began reading out the statement.

"Cut and fry the onions in butter. Place fried onions in turkey and cook it."

"Ehhh that doesn't sound right," Jennifer said.

Sue vigorously shook her head up and down.

"That's how I cooked it." Sue typed out.

Jennifer proceeded to fry the onions in butter, and placed the onions in the roaster with the turkey.

I returned home from work and as soon as I entered the house it smelt amazing and I was ready to dig in. Once a year, Sue always treated us to her mother's delicious homemade dressing recipe which consisted of frying onions in butter, and placing the onions in the bread before baking it. You can imagine my shock when I walked over to the roaster and saw onions mixed in with the turkey. Suddenly I saw as Jennifer slapped her forehead.

"Oh no," she said.

"What the heck is this?" I asked.

She looked at Sue and began pointing.

"She tricked me I swear she told me to do it." Jennifer said.

"You told me to include her in making it and I did. She told me to put the onions with the turkey. I completely spaced on the fact that it was supposed to go in the dressing."

We both simultaneously looked at Sue who had suddenly bust into a hysterical laugh. She laughed so hard she would stop mid laugh taking in a deep croak sounding of breath.

"Sue did you tell her to do that?" I asked.

Sue shook her head in a motion of "No" while shrieking in between breaths. I walked over and looked at the computer where the words from the day remained. Just as Jennifer had indicated Sue had told her to place the onions in the turkey. It was obvious that Sue had purposefully sabotaged Thanksgiving dinner. We didn't dwell on it much though. Sue had her laughs which made it worthwhile. It was obvious at times she liked to torture us with her antics. She had a good laugh and we went about our day trying to celebrate Thanksgiving like any other family.

The holiday gave us the opportunity to escape from the daily grind of life that consisted of doctors, hospitals and various other medical emergencies. They were lonely times though. No one came around on holidays. No help came. 911 was there but that was all the help one can get on a holiday. And if the holidays is on a Friday and Monday then most of that week is without help coming into the home. Holidays are bitter sweet to say the least.

Sue was obviously slipping away. Her skin was tough like leather, and face retracted leaving an outline of bones. We went back to the MS clinic and met with Dr. Castro.

"We want to try an experimental drug." The doctor said, "We want her to go on Methotrexate infusion."

Methotrexate was a chemotherapy drug. My Insurance Company inquired why we were requesting coverage for a drug for a person who didn't have cancer. It leads to a four month fight that I let the doctors and Insurance Company work out themselves. While at the clinic I rolled Sue into an elevator with another woman.

"What does she have?" She asked.

"Either MS or a breakdown of the central nervous system. Not really sure." I replied.

"I used to be like her but I take the infusion now." She said.

She looked for lack of a better word, normal, nothing in comparison to how Sue looked. It gave us great hope. Hope however, is a scary thing, especially for someone like Sue. Throughout her whole ordeal she never lost hope and I never quite understood how.

I received a call from UT Southwestern giving me a date and time to bring Sue to Zales Hospital on The UT Southwestern campus in Dallas. At the end of November 2010 we got Sue dressed and loaded up to travel to Zales Hospital. We checked in, signed my life away and got her into the bed.

A doctor later entered the room.

"You are doing a great job taking care of her. It shows that you are doing a great job." He said. "Thank You." I replied.

(The doctor said that to me because of The 911 packet. I would take the packet to the hospital. The doctor could see all the information that I include into a packet. They would scan the 911 packet and all who needs to see the information could see all the important information. Please look for The 911 packet in Chapter 8. Later on, I fully explained the 911 packet better in my second book, Caregiving: How to Set up Caregiving in the Home).

The hospital staff drew blood and urine from Sue and returned to the room about an hour later the same doctor came in and told us, "I'm sorry we can't do the infusion. She has a urinary tract infection. Here is a prescription, take her home and come back in ten days." As I got her dressed and loaded in the car and while driving us back to the house I wondered, *if I was ever going to know if this drug would help her.*

A majority of Sue's medication was mixed together with her nutritional supplement meal. If her medication was in pill form, the pills were crushed and poured into the container, before being administered through her G-Tube. Due to Sue's swallowing difficulty every attempt was made not to force her to try and swallow pills.

Some medication however, could not be broken or smashed to be administered via G-Tube. In these types of situations the easiest way was to place the pill in a spoonful of yogurt, followed by a drink in order to get the medicine into her body.

Every day was spent feeding, showering, brushing her teeth, giving medication, changing medication, taking her to doctors, running to get prescriptions, running from one end of the house to the next, taking on the next fight. It was daily and each day was demanding, and every day felt like a never ending Monday. It was anguishing to work and administrate her care. It was hard to deal with the IRS, the Insurance Company and spending issues. It was not a cheap experience to delve into in a home setting. It was quite expensive and we were far away from all of Sue's doctors. Each and every day, over and over we administered Sue's care.

Care giving had become *Our Labor of Love*. Even the most loving person can crumble under the stress of an enormous undertaking such as this. It pushed me to the brink and brought me crashing back down to Earth each time. Sure there were blessings to be had for Sue and I, although those blessings felt few and far between. There was a website I discovered called Caregiver Action Network. It was a good place for me to go in times of need to know I was not alone in my undertaking. Not to mention it gave me the opportunity to vent when I needed to. I was able to say what I needed to say, and obtain advice from others Souls who had gone before me. I needed advice countless times, and I did not know anyone personally who was remotely close to going through what I was going through. Here is the *About Us* on their web site:

"The Caregiver Action Network is the nation's leading family caregiver organization working to improve the quality of life for the more than 90 million Americans who care for loved ones with chronic conditions, disabilities, disease, or the frailties of old age. CAN serves a broad spectrum of family caregivers ranging from the parents of children with special needs, to the families and friends of wounded soldiers; from a young couple dealing with a diagnosis of MS, to adult children caring for parents with Alzheimer's disease. CAN (formerly the National Family Caregivers Association) is a non-profit organization providing education, peer support, and resources to family caregivers across the country free of charge."

http://www.caregiveraction.org/

Sue had a *depilation of her immune system*. I felt isolated from my congregation and was becoming increasingly frustrated that I was receiving very little assistance from my church. And then it dawned on me, I did not want church members or anyone for that matter entering our home if they were sick. I had often discouraged visitors from entering our home. In fact the first thing you saw when you came to our house was a sign on the front door:

If you have a cold, if you are sick, if you are running a fever please do not enter my home.

Yet, there were so many Home Medical and other professionals who came into my home sick, contaminating the residence with their coughing, strep throat and even the flu. I thank God for allowing me to see it was me and not His Church, and immediately asked God for forgiveness. We would have been truly blessed had I allowed the Church to come into our home.

Captains at work were handing me counseling cards. They were quietly telling me to get some help. I was afraid of counseling and I was afraid of opening up to anyone regarding our situation. I learned things as I continued to struggle though. There were times I cried out because I could not take one more thing added to my load. Yet, I kept on going and attempting to strive every day. Each day was a new sacrifice in care giving. It is crazy, it is maddening, and it is something I had never done before. Caregiving was one of the hardest, demanding places I had ever been in my life. It was difficult to say the least to see my wife dying slowly in front of my eyes. It was gut wrenching, and heart breaking. I slowly came to the realization that I would one day live on, and Sue would not. I kept caring for her as though she would be healed.

I was so demanding on my family, doctors, politicians, and pharmacies. I became Sue's Advocate, because no one else could or would. As Sue lost her ability in every aspect I had to be there to ensure her every day bodily functions operated with assistance. A common definition I began to hear and experience firsthand was *Activities of Daily Living* (ADLs). I Goggle ADL:

"The term "activities of daily living," or ADLs, refers to the basic tasks of everyday life, such as eating, bathing, dressing, toileting, and transferring. When people are unable to perform these activities, they need help in order to cope, either from other human beings or mechanical devices or both."

https://www.google.com/#q=Activities+of+Daily+Living

This is when the fight for Sue really kicked in for she became helpless. Sue needed help with everything, regardless of the toll it took on me. The constant transferring of Sue from one place to another such as the scooter to the hospital bed caused a rip in my right knee. I additionally developed arthritis in my left knee. I eventually became so exhausted I almost checked myself into a hospital.

Caregiving began to change me in unimaginable ways. "I want you to kill me please!" Sue asks me, hinting at various prospects in the ways she could die. Not only mentioning it to me, but to Jennifer and Travis as well. Slowly, and inevitably she asked me to end her life. She was struggling to grasp life as one day possibly bedridden, a shell of a person. I secretly mulled over the prospect of continuing life without the love of my life. I debated with myself the consequences of those actions, and thought to myself if it were ever to happen I would be leaving this world with her. The anger, and sadness was overbearing and I had no one to console me through my issues. After hearing of Sue's initial request I thought about trying to move us to Oregon. Oregon is one of the few states in America that has laws in relation to Death with Dignity. Oregon law requires living in the state, and gaining residency status in order to obtain the prescribed drugs to end your life on your terms. Our finances were still essentially "shot" and I could not afford the move. Not to mention losing Insurance during this time for Sue would ultimately lead to more suffering while awaiting the residency status. In order to understand Sue's thought process for her request you have to understand the tumultuous and overwhelming pain she endured. Her 1981 car wreck paled in comparison to a medical issue that couldn't be cured, or really even treated.

The stress was taking its toll on us all. One month I noticed I was starting to lose weight, the unexplained weight loss made me fear for my own health. My time was completely depleted at work and I was in danger of "falling of the books" As a Correctional Officer under a state government agency, once all of my compensation: holiday, vacation, overtime, and sick time was depleted I could technically still not come to work. However, once the time ran out obviously I would not be paid days taken off. The worst part of "falling off the books" was the paycheck which was normally available on the first day of the month would not be given until the 15th of the month. This scenario was one of my worst fears, as I could not imagine waiting an additional two weeks for a paycheck in the midst of caring for Sue.

There were days that I was so tired I could not even brush my teeth. There were nights I was so tired I could not sleep. I was getting only an hour of uninterrupted sleep when I lay down before being awaken to Sue wanting something. Caregiving and working full time was such a struggle. My back was against the wall and I did not know how I was going to make it or how I could do much more than I was already doing for Sue. I had to start finding out ways to ease up my load of stress that was building up in me.

I was driving home one day from work. It was late since I slowed down my driving speed. I drove sixty miles per hour coming home. Due to I knew it was on in caregiving, when I got home. I got up at 3 A.M. Took care of Sue until 4:30 A.M. and then drove to work and worked 8:45 hours a day. I used to back in those days spend three hundred and fifty dollars a month in gas just going to work. I found by driving sixty miles an hour I cut my gas bill in half to one hundred and seventy five dollars a month now.

I started seeing billboards on I-45 North and South bound and found blessings on a billboard ministry stationed out of Springfield, Missouri from Assemblies of God Church Headquarters. I had found five large billboards during my commute to work. One of these billboards was in my small town and had lights on it that lit the billboard up like high noon throughout the night. I left for work around 4:30 A.M. and that sign was there. Regardless of if I went North or South, or if I left and came home and day or night on the highway, I would see those billboards every day.

The billboard revealed, a man setting on the floor with his back against the wall. His knees were bent up and his elbows were on his knees with his face buried in his hands. The captions said,

All Things are Possible with God.

That was me on that billboard. I had my back against the wall in at home and work. I did not have the energy to work. I did not have energy to care. I looked at that sign over and over. I read that caption over and over and I told God,

"My back is against the wall; how can I do this Lord? How can I know all things are possible when all things are impossible? How can I get off that billboard? How can I find what You want from me? How Lord can I get back upon my feet?"

Over and over as I went to work and came back to work there was that billboard. I looked at all five of them billboards every day for over six months or more. Only God can use something such as a billboard to bless a tired Child of His.

God is so good to us, I thought.

I did not know how to go forward. I was lost and unsure of when life would feel some normality again. All I knew was God was in control. I would ask God why?

Why Lord at her young age did we have this come into our lives? Why in 1981 did you give us a miracle just to take that miracle away from us now?" Even holidays did not feel the same any more.

CHAPTER EIGHT

Looking for Help

I was in dire need of a new at Home healthcare worker. My time was low and Jennifer was leaving. This left me with very little options. I knew I needed to work in order to build up more time for emergencies. I opened up my home again and began calling the list of sitters. Word got out and people began to call or come to our house due to interest in the job. During the interviews I found myself in the same predicament as last time. One woman came into our home, and I explained the job requirements, as well as the little perks I could offer. I explained the Unemployment Insurance, Workman's Compensation and how I offered time off for designated pre-approved days. Pre-approved days were essential because I needed to be able to take off of work in order to cover the day. A black woman came into my home for an interview.

"Would you let a Mexican lady work for you and pay her under another name?" She asked.

"No I said that's illegal." I replied.

"Would you let a Mexican man come and work under a different name?"

"No." I replied. I told her we did not need her services and showed her the door.

It was very frustrating looking for a new employee. I needed someone honest, forthright, and hardworking people. I didn't want someone who was going to jeopardize my freedom for a few extra dollars. We ended up hiring a young woman, I wanted to employ her mother but Sue wanted her daughter. "I do not want the mother she cannot lift me," Sue said to me.

I took a couple of weeks off at the prison in order to train her in my home. During the training I had to take Sue to the hospital. After the trip to the hospital I took Sue home and returned to town to fill her prescription, I had approximately fifteen dollars to my name.

"Ok that will be thirty five dollars Mr. Patterson." The customer service woman behind the pharmacy counter said.

"All I have is fifteen dollars!" I cried out.

I walked back to my car in shame. I swore from that day on I would never run out of money again. Regardless of our situation Sue always had to have the things she needed. I had to wait five days for the first of the month to get that prescription for Sue. Despite what anyone says there were times I had to overdraw my account. My bank covered up to five hundred dollars on overdraft protection. When the 1st of the month did not fall on my days off then I would go to town and get our food and our medicine and suffer with a thirty five dollar overdraft fee later. It simply made the stress less by not having to go do all the grocery buying on a day that I worked and had to come home to caregiving.

Sue had no complaints with our new employee which was rare for her. Everything seemed ok and for a time I felt like life may finally start to settle down.

To assist the new employee in Sue's care I put bulletins and packets on the door and walls. How to deal with Sue if you are confused in how to care for her:

Call 911 for Police or Ambulance. For a poison emergency in the United States call 800-222-1222, call my insurance RN nurse @ 877-731-****. Call the doctor on Call for DR Youngblood @ 972-875-****.

Call for health questions @ 866-336-**** Policy number and group number, and or call John Patterson at work with my number.

Additionally attached to the wall was our 911 packet for hospital trips. Included in the packet was information regarding Sue such as: full name, birth date, height, weight, and a list of allergies. It listed daily medications, notice of Sue's G-Tube and how it was cared for. As well as contact information for the primary Doctor, and specialists in Urology and Neurology. It also listed her possible diagnose from all doctors. I was listed as Sue's agent and enclosed were the Power of Attorneys with copies. Then the last thing on this document was what to do when Sue passed on. It gave the number for body pick up through UT Southwestern and provided a copy of the body will document. This 911 document went with us to Hospitals, to Doctors and to Clinics. Essentially the packet was for anyone who might need information on Sue and her current condition. Doctors and intake people would take possession of the packet, preventing further redundant questioning.

I was at home with Sue when a Home health nurse came into our home.

"I am going to fill out this Medicaid application while you tend to Sue." I said

It was no problem. I had filled out so many applications looking for some kind of help. I had the application filled out before the visit was over with.

"That is done now I can send it off." I said.

"You got that filled out all ready?" The home nurse asked me.

When I first tried asking for help it would take hours and hours to fill out the required paperwork. I was so use to the mounds of paperwork that came with caring for Sue that a Medicaid application became a cake walk. Sue was already a recipient of Medicare due to her lingering disability associated with the 1981 car wreck. The reason I was attempting to obtain the Medicaid was to help alleviate some of the cost associated with Sue's care.

All of Sue's income from disability went into covering the costs of trips to the Doctors, Co pays, Prescriptions and Hospitalizations. My income was solely dedicated to paying our bills. I was trying to keep a two income household afloat on one income.

I sent the application to Medicaid in the mail and a month later I received the denial letter stating that we did not qualify. I called the number on the back with the intent of having an Appeal. I spoke with an intake worker regarding the Appeal.

"Yes we make more than $2,000 a month. But, if you would look at what I pay out throughout the month for health care costs you will find that we do not make $2,000 a month." I said.

I had to explain myself six times before she understood what I was saying. I was informed they would be calling me to set up a time for court. A few days later I went to Jean DeWald in Dallas. We went over the paperwork for four hours.

"John what do you really want here?" She asked.

"I just want to show on paper that I've exhausted my means." I replied.

In May of 2011 I received a letter informing me I needed to call a number on a certain date for my Appeal. I awoke that morning and called the number. They put me on hold while awaiting the conference call to begin. Included in the Appeal was a Judge, a Represented from the Texas Department of Health and Human Services and myself.

"Mr. Patterson your lawyer has not shown up. Do you want a continuance or do you want to argue for your wife?" The Judge asked.

"I will argue for my wife thank you." I replied.

The Judge explained the process to me and stated the Representative for the State would go first. I was informed to not interrupt her while she presented her testimony and evidence.

"When she is done I will give you a chance for rebuttal." The Judge stated.

"That is fine." I replied.

"No, No, No, No. I gave him a 165 page report and showed them they did not qualify. I gave him a $20 credit off the $2,000 a month," said the State Representative.

No, No, No for 45 minutes she said No before there was finally silence.

"Do you have any questions about her evidence or testimony?" Asked the Judge?

"No I do not." I replied.

"Ok it is your turn Mr. Patterson to give your testimony and evidence." The Judge stated.

"Let's look at this 165 page report and turn to my plea. Yes I make more than $2,000 a month but if you would look at my expenses throughout the month you would find that we do not make $2,000 a month." I said.

To prove my expenses I provided evidence of my 2010 1040 A, IRS tax document.

"You see our adjusted gross is $34,000. Now look at line 40, the deductions. You see that $24,000, that is medical related. Now look toward the bottom you will see I was supposed to pay $3,500 this year. Do you see that dark line toward the bottom, look down under that dark line and you will see what I really paid in taxes which is $350. This $350 is 10% of my tax burden this year. Under that dark line is all the people who made less than $2,000 a month. They were taxed 10% not the regular tax that everyone else paid." I said to them.

"Are you finished with your testimony and evidence?" The Judge asked.

"Yes." I replied.

The Judge ask the State Resprenstive if she wanted a chance for rebuttal on my testimony or evidence, in which she replied,

"No."

"I will rule in August," said the Judge.

I heard a gasp from what I assume was the Representative for the State. I knew we had a long wait in store for us.

In July of 2011 Sue started to complain about her butt being sore. We started placing pillows under one side to take pressure off her bottom. We traveled to the Hospital twice, once because of a leaking Foley. They kept her for twenty four hours to see if she suffered a stroke. After being released we were back a few days later due to a blockage in her rectum. It hurt me to see Sue be treated like this due to her blockage in her rectum. I held Sue down while the Physician Assistance reach up into Sue to pull the blockage out.

I did not want to take Sue to a hospital again for this kind experience which led me having to track her bowel movements from now on in the journal. That way we never again went to the hospital to have Sue go through that kind of treatment ever again. If she did not have a bowel movement in seventy two hours then I would react by giving her Magnesium Citrate, Top down and or an Enema, Bottom up.

We went to an Urologist at UT Southwestern. Sue was having problem with leakage of the bladder, otherwise known as Incontinence. The Urologists placed a Suprapubic Catheter into Sue. This is a surgery where a hole is drilled into the bladder and a tube is inserted that attaches to a Foley catheter. This is considered a more long term solution compared to regular catheters which have to be changed regularly. Catheters additionally have greater risk of infection. Sue had two of these Suprapubic Catheters surgically inserted none of which took properly. The first one did not work right and was later replaced by the Urologist. The day after the second surgery I rushed Sue back to a local hospital due to huge amount of blood in her urine bag. The ER doctor put a Foley back into her urethra and sent us home with a Suprapubic Catheter and a Foley inserted into her urethra. Sue was forced to keep both types of catheters in for a week until the Suprapubic Catheter could be removed.

We were required to get an order from UT Southwestern to take her to the local hospital and pull out the Suprapubic Catheter. The doctors determined that Sue was one of the rare patients whose bladder healed improperly within the first twenty four hours of the surgery. This prevented the urine from exiting the bladder, and explained why only blood was entering the urine collection bag. After the two failed attempts despite the risk associated with a Foley catheter, Sue and I decided not to attempt the Suprapubic Catheter again. I got a letter from the Urologist department near the end of caregiving. The letter was a survey that said our records show you have had a Suprapubic Catheter placed in. I checked the, "It did not help" box and sent it back to them.

Finally at the end of August 2011, I received a letter from Medicaid, and from the Texas Health and Human Services Commission:

The information presented during you appeal hearing has been carefully considered, and the original decision has been SUSTAINED.

I called them because I honestly did not understand how their original decision was upheld. I had such high hopes that this ruling could have shaken up the $2,000 rule that most States and the US government hold. If the Judge had ruled in my favor it would have sent shock waves throughout the system.

I looked everywhere within the United States government for help. I simply could not get past the $2,000 rule. I called United Way, and was told they couldn't help me. I was mainly told to seek assistance from churches; but even they were struggling due to the state of the economy that the United states was in.

I was determined to only ask my church as a last resort. On a Wednesday night a brother from my church came up to me and shook my hand, and left a hundred dollar bill in my hand. My church was helping as they could by giving me two hundred dollars here and two hundred dollars there. When I attended church which was not very often due to the constraints of caregiving I would generally sit in the back. It was hard to sing God's praises knowing my wife was home dying.

As soon as the service was over I would be the first one out the door so I could get home faster to Sue. One day a brother ran after me as I was starting my car. He knocked on my window, startling me, and handed me four hundred dollars. I was shocked and told him thank you rather quickly. I still do not know who that brother was as I did not get a good look at him. In caregiving there is not much money; most of your money goes to the care. I felt like I was working every minute of every hour of every day, three hundred and sixty five days a year. I felt as though I was alone, and that no one was there to help. I especially felt as if no one was experiencing what we were in our lives. That is not true; there are plenty of people doing care giving. I found out on that caregiving site I used.

Sue and I actually lived on prayer, one day at a time. Before Sue became ill there were certain things I just did not do around the house. I never did dishes, cooked, cleaned, or really took care of anything. I came home like most men from a job, thinking that once I was home my duties were done for the day. Sue being a stay at home wife handled everything in the household; therefore I took this time to relax the best I could. I'm not sure if I was more unprepared for the caregiving, or for my adjustment without her.

I planned out my care by researching the illness. In my case there were so many different systems of illness that I spent many hours in research. Research in some ways made me better prepared for the progression of her disease. This was part of what fueled our planning for the future. Hard, life ending decisions had to be made, and Sue and I made these decisions during a time we were equipped to do so.

The most important thing to never neglect outside of your love one, is you, something I sometimes forgot about. I over exhausted myself many a times. It took me a long time to remember to take time out for myself. I finally got to the point where I allowed people I trusted to come into our home to take care of Sue so I could do something as simple as go to a two hour movie, or eat at a restaurant. It was nice, but when I headed home the sinking feeling of being a caregiver would set in again. In the restaurant I ate alone. Something I never had to do before, I would look at other families and wonder to myself, *Wow if families only knew how precious family members are?*

Despite the exhaustion it was imperative to press on as a caregiver. Regardless of how I felt, and the turmoil I was experiencing I knew it paled in comparison to how Sue felt. It was vital to hold the highest level of care possible to Sue, and to never toe the line of neglect. There is never any room whatsoever for abusive behavior towards a loved one regardless of the situation. There is never any room in caregiving for Abuse! BEST REMBER THAT OR YOU GO TO JAIL!

I was at work one morning, and was giving breaks to other officers on various buildings.

"Where is Officer Patterson?" The captain said over the radio.

"Patterson on Echo building breaking." I called out on the radio. I repeated over and over on the radio while it was obvious he couldn't hear me as he continually asked,

"Where is Officer Patterson?"

Finally he heard me respond on the radio and he immediately called the Shift Lieutenant for a relief officer to my location. The officer who relieved me directed me to the Human Resource office in the Administration Building near the front lobby. After being relieved I started the long walk to the Administration Building. I walked the walkway referred to as the "slab", or the "bowling alley." The slab has painted yellow lines running parallel to one another from one end of the prison to the other. Officers walk the slab while offenders walk the yellow lines on the edge of the slab. Located at various portions of the slab is what is referred to as crash gates. A crash gate is a fence with a door, the door was locked or open, by a key or by a control room. I walked past crash gates, offenders, and Correctional Officers and felt the eyes of everyone upon me.

While I waited at the last crash gates for the familiar buzz of the door unlocking I feared for what news was awaiting me at the end of the walk. I sensed the prison would not let me have a direct line in case the call was a death notice call. I think everyone was on edge, and slightly worried how I would handle Sue's death should she pass while I was at work.

When I walked into Human Resource office there stood my Lieutenant standing over a phone off the hook. I picked up the phone feeling dreadful.

"Hello?" I asked.

"Sue called the police and now I think she needs to go to the hospital," said my home care worker.

"Grab the 911 packet off the wall and call 911 and go with her to the hospital. After work I will pick you two up and take you home." I stated.

My health care worker had laid her cell phone on the desk with Sue. Sue knowing dialing 911 was part of her fun with people seeing how they handle emergency in the home with her. Sue called the police. Since she was unable to speak anymore there was nothing but silence on the phone. The police called the house and the worker did not know how to handle the situation and immediately called the prison looking for guidance.

Situations like these were becoming frequent. I had inkling that our second care worker was feeling the stress of our situation. Taking care of Sue was an exhausting job and a couple of hours a day for several days could make you tired beyond belief. The second employee resigned her position on April 15, 2011. It appeared I was going to have to try and find someone to take care of Sue as quickly as possible.

CHAPTER NINE

All in the Family

After the worker left I requested leave from the Family Medical Leave Act (FMLA) and was granted my leave. The ordeal of searching for a new employee had ensued yet again, and I felt overburdened yet again. On April 23, 2011 during my search our son Travis called me. He told me he could come down and help if I wanted him to. I offered to pay him what I would pay anyone else working in our house, taking care of Sue. Travis packed up his car and drove down to Texas from Missouri about a week later. He had officially moved back to take care of his ailing mother and offered to receive two hundred dollars less a month to free up money for bills. Despite saving me weeks of searching for a new employee I still had to continue FMLA in order to train Travis on Sue's lengthy schedule.

Travis was about to encounter what Jennifer had already experience, the unpleasant and awkward moments that occur within caregiving. Bathing, dressing, and toiletry are just some of the duties a child can be unaccustomed to performing for an ailing parent. I knew it was a shock for Jennifer the first time she bathed Sue, but she was gradually eased into the situation as Sue declined. Travis would not be afforded that luxury, and would be thrown into Sue's current state.

Shortly after arriving Travis awoke to an assortment of bites all over his body. Travis was highly allergic to several things including most insects, spiders, and fleas.

"Oh crap. I let the last employee sleep on that mattress with her dog," I said.

"Well I think I'm going to need a new mattress." Travis replied as he reached behind his back to scratch.

The second employee would sometimes stay at our house early in the morning in case of an emergency. I could not afford to pay her for extra hours to start as soon as I left our house for work. Our employee would sometimes stay the night and would sometimes come in early and rest a couple of hours before work. I allowed her to bring her dog in and without realizing it the mattress had become infested with fleas.

I went to town that day and was fearful the entire drive. Because of how recent my Bankruptcy was, I was unsure of whether or not I would be able to qualify for any type of loan or credit for a new mattress. I learned a hard lesson that day after I found a mattress company that did not do a credit check loan; a type of loan. Unfortunately as desperately as we needed the mattress I would end up paying three times what the mattress was worth.

In May 2011 we received a call from Hospice.

"Are you ready for us to enter your life?" The caller asked.

"I am waiting to see what happens with the chemo we are doing first before we make any decisions." I replied.

At Christmas 2011 a preacher in a Methodist church preached to his flock the true meaning of Christmas aside from a tree and presents. He preached about bringing blessings upon others, other than, spending money for gifts. There was a man in the church who knew about our struggles. He called upon his Sunday School to adopt our family for the Christmas. I assumed a Sunday School could not do much in the way of giving. He called me one afternoon to tell me they had a check for Sue and I. I told him I would meet him half way, and we settled on Whataburger restaurant right off the highway. He handed me an eleven hundred dollar check, and I was blown away by their generosity.

"My Church members do not necessarily venture out to perform their ministry but instead they find those who need assistance and assisted them." My friend said to me.

People I knew, and others that I did not know, came together to help Sue and I. One day someone gave me two hundred dollars, and then a man sent a check for one thousand dollars.

At some point I finally got an answer from the letter I wrote to the Honorable Joe Barton. When I sent the letter to The Honorable Congressmen Joe Barton and he started an insurance inquiry, which caused my Insurance Company to send the claim from their office to Employee Retirement System (ERS). ERS is responsible for State of Texas employees, and oversees several state employee benefits such as insurance and retirement. ERS email me and informed me that they would not accept our Power of Attorney. I immediately loaded Sue in the car and took her to the bank. ERS had sent in the email the Power of Attorney they wanted notarized. We get to the bank and I knew the biggest hurdle of this new ordeal would delve from Sue's inability to write.

"Can she make an X?" I asked the notary at the bank because it is what I had always seen done in the movies.

She grabbed the phone and called the home office.

"Let's see how well she can sign." She said as she handed me a pen and scrap paper.

On a practice paper Sue surprisingly did pretty well with her signature. But when it came to signing the actual document, it looked like a 2-year-old could have written it out better. The lady at the bank notarized the Power of Attorney and I sent it back to ERS by mail and fax. I wrote a letter to ERS explaining to them how we had to insert a G-tube into my wife's stomach wall. It was required for her survival and medical necessary. My Insurance

Company refused to pay for the life sustaining protein shakes. I waited for a couple of days and then I called ERS to see the status of the paperwork.

"Did you get my fax on the Power of Attorney for my wife Sue Patterson?" I asked.

"Yes. Your letter has spurred us into action!" She replied.

"Oh really? What are you going to do?" I said.

"We just got this give us some time." She said.

ERS sent the paperwork to a higher level in my Insurance Company to investigate why the Dallas office did not pay my original claim. A person from Abilene, Texas later called me. She apologized for the run around that I had received and said that the claim would be getting paid.

My Insurance Company was wrong to tell me the little they paid was all they were going to pay. What my Insurance Company did was teach me just how insurance works. Every time I made a claim the first answer was always "No." I am sure most people just accept that first no and move on. I did not and I appealed their decision not to pay me. I learned that when I called my Insurance Company they keep a record of reference numbers, and it is important to request and keep that reference number. I learned the most important two words insurance wants to hear "Medically Necessary." I learned that when you order supplies associated with Incontinence, bladder leakage, Foleys you need two more words that produce much supply, Supply me with what "Medicaid allows." I learned you can Appeal any decision, and if the insurance refuses the Appeal then you can Appeal even further as I did outside of my Insurance Company and inside in my case ERS. I felt as though I was playing a game of whack-a-mole. Every time one problem settled two more problems appeared, and sometimes those problems were detrimental.

I took Sue to the hospital yet again when I saw her mouth was crooked. An acronym I had learned a long time ago to help identify strokes referred to as FAST help me realize something was wrong with Sue. FAST stands for: Facial drooping, Arm weakness, Speech difficulties, and Time. Sue started to have mini strokes in her brain referred to as Transient Ischemic Attacks (TIA), as the doctors diagnosed it. It did some minor damage to her brain at that time.

A couple of weeks later UT Southwestern called me again. I was told to bring Sue to the Aston building of the hospital which was the transplant unit. The floor mainly dealt with patients who were receiving an assortment of various transplants. Patients on this floor who were receiving transplants most often were given a drug called Methotrexate. This was the same drug the doctors were planning to give Sue experimentally. The drug was also generally used for cancer patients, which is obviously not what Sue was suffering from. Because of her fragile state, the doctors thought Sue being on this floor would suit her better with staff who was accustomed to administrating the drug.

We admitted her on August 8, 2011 and I felt like I was signing my life away again before taking her to her room. This time the doctor put a lot of antibiotic's into her IV to flush her system. This hospital was a teaching hospital. They used our family to teach their students while we were there. Person after person were brought into our room including countless doctors, nurses, and various professionals. Every time a lead doctor entered hordes of what I can only assume were Resident's would follow.

"Would you give this patient, Mrs. Patterson a Methotrexate infusion?" A doctor would ask. Some would nod in agreement while others would vehemently shake their heads no.

"She's too far gone." One would say.

"She would not make it." Another would say.

It became apparent that some of the doctors were arguing over whether or not the drug itself would kill Sue. I began to fear the infusion due to the widening negative connotations I heard uttered every time a new group of doctors entered our room. We were assigned an Intern to our case which was an extra benefit I felt because she continually explained and expanded on what little the doctors said. Around 9 P.M. they took Sue and I to another room. The Intern came in and read to us all the things that could go wrong over the course of thirty minutes. There were many possibilities of nasty side effect that ultimately could harm or kill Sue. Dr. Castro came in soon after the reading, and they handed me the consent forms.

"If you sign here we will do the infusion." The Intern stated.

I took the pen and signed it *Sue Ann Patterson, John Patterson, POA*. Dr. Castro took the paper and she signed it as well. They brought in an IV bag containing the drug with a coal black bag covering it. The Methotrexate was a beautiful greenish color but even florescent light could cause the drug to break down, hence the cover. They put the drug into her IV and Sue and I sat there and watched *All in the Family*, laughing as the Methotrexate coursed through her veins.

I fell asleep around 2 A.M. and awoke at 5 A.M. to hordes of medical staff assembling into our room. I shook their hands and I introduced Sue to them.

"Oh I know Mrs. Patterson," said one Doctor.

He had been up all night seeing the transfusion. I looked at Sue and observed her once pale, almost lifeless skin looked healthy on her face and hands. She looked stronger, and I thought this was nothing short of a miracle.

Oh I prayed, *"Lord let this be!"*

She still had to stay in the hospital for another few days. Everyone that came into our room was beautiful towards us.

"What are you doing here this is the time for you to go get rest, while we will take care of her," said a staff member.

I found whenever Sue was at the hospital I never left. However, when I really did need a rest Travis or Jennifer would come to the hospital and essentially camp out with Sue. None of us ever wanted her to be alone, surrounded by strangers. Besides no one understood just how demanding she could be. When Sue wanted something like a Chap Stick she was going to get it or you were going to be miserable.

There were many times on trips like this one that I would bring all of her medication and demand to be one that gave it to her. Sue had a rigorous course of prescriptions mainly geared towards Pain Management, Digestive needs, and Neurological needs. Generally the Nurses would enter and attempt to confiscate all of her medication despite my requests to keep the medicine and do it myself. I understood they had their own logs to fill in order to keep track of what was occurring and when it was occurring. But no one knew Sue the way I did, and no one knew her schedule like I did. It was important to always keep the medications on schedule.

"John you cannot keep these drugs in here you have to let the nurse take my drugs and they will give them back to us when we go home," Sue typed out to me.

On this occasion I was finally able to negotiate a compromise where the nurses would bring me the medication directly at its scheduled time and I would administer it myself. Many times I went to the RN desk and requested medicine for Sue to keep Sue on the schedule.

Each time we knew there was a hospital visit looming I packed a bag and collected one hundred dollars. I referred to it as going camping. I would camp out in Sue's hospital room and continue on with her care. If I went home and rested, it would have to take months to bring her back to the level of care where we were giving Sue before the hospital trip. It just was not worth all the work to get Sue back on track so I could go get some rest while she was in the hospital.

"I'm here to help and care for her the way I know but not get into your way," I would say each time I met a new nurse. I let them do everything but her feedings, and her medication administration.

Jennifer drove two and half hours to the hospital to keep me company, and stopped along the way to pick up Travis. It helped pass the time.

After the infusion I overheard a conversation between two doctors.

"She is the second female that has positive results with this infusion." He said.

We went home with hope and joy! Sue was delighted which shines through on the picture used as the cover for this book. You can see the hope in her eyes and the smile of life. Prior to the transfusion a Peripherally Inserted Central Catheter (PICC line) was placed in her chest because her veins were too small and there was a fear they were too weak to support the infusion. A PICC line generally is positioned near a large central vein that directly drains near the heart.

After returning home a home health care nurse entered our home a few days later in order to properly clean Sue's PICC line. While I watched her clean I looked closely to see what was being done.

"Can you teach me once you're done so that I know how to clean it?" I asked.

"Oh no." She said shaking her head somewhat startled, "We can't do that, you're not trained for that."

In hindsight the doctor knew that I needed to also know how to clean the PICC line, as the Methotrexate was involved in an ongoing treatment plan. The treatment plan was expected to continue for six months to a year depending on how Sue responded. The doctor and I both knew that home health care nurses would not be available every time the PICC line needed to be cleaned. The Doctor provided me with a "standing order" stating I needed to be taught how to clean the PICC line. Luckily I had the order readily available, filed away awaiting the arrival of this moment. I reached into the drawer and located the standing order handing it to the nurse. She looked it over for a moment, and quickly called who I could only assume was her supervisor with the order.

"He's got an order from the doctor saying he needs to be taught how to clean her PICC line." The nurse said.

I waited patiently as she continued the conversation on the phone.

"Can you make a copy of the order for me to take back with me?" She asked.

"Of course." I replied as I turned on the copier, and made the copy.

After all was said and done the nurse began to go over the details of how to clean the PICC line. The PICC line was one of the most complicated things we dealt with during Sue's care. When cleaning the PICC line you had to be sure not to touch the syringe insert areas with bare fingers, as well as they could not touch Sue's skin, and they could not touch one another. After cleaning the inserts a dose of Heparin (an anti-coagulant) had to be administered in order to prevent blood clots from forming.

Just as we felt the hope wash over us when arriving home it dissipated almost immediately. While I was watching the news they began discussing the drug Methotrexate. They said the drug was going Generic and that the Food and Drug Administration closed down the only plant that made the drug in the United States due to production problems.

"No!!" I cried out.

The news report continued saying Methotrexate was the best possible treatment for children with certain cancer. It appeared their lives, and Sue's was in jeopardy. A few days later I received a phone call from UT Southwestern.

"We are sorry. We can't get the drug now. If you want when we get supplies that are left over we could make that available for your wife. If you're ok with that," The woman stated.

"Yes, we will take what we can get." I replied.

Supply's left over from my understanding at the time meant that we had to wait for a transplant person or a person with cancer to pass away, and then their supply would go to us. As was explained to me, when a treatment plan was set with a patient a full order was placed for however much of the drug was needed for the rest of the treatment plan. As heart wrenching, and morbid as it was, it was the only option available for us at the time. The Doctor put Sue on Cell Cept, a drug similar to Methotrexate.

The Cell Cept came in liquid form unlike the Methotrexate meaning we no longer had any use for the PICC line. Our local hospital initially refused to remove the PICC line without an order from UT Southwestern. I contacted UT Southwestern and was luckily able to obtain the order for it to be removed, and it was removed. All of the several months of hard work seemed to have been for absolutely nothing.

We would have to go every month for six months to test her blood levels since she was taking Cell Cept. I told UT Southwestern that I wanted to do it in a local hospital as it was nine miles round trip compared to one hundred fifty miles for every trip to UT Southwestern. They agreed and gave us a Standing Order for a year at our local hospital. I made copies and took them to the hospital and admitted Sue. That way each month we would take her to the lab for the blood test associated with Cell Cept.

Of course nothing was ever easy when it came to Sue's care and the lab seemed confused about the standing order. The order stated that all lab paperwork was to be faxed to UT Southwestern. I was forced to go to records and ask them for a copy of the labs each time because the lab never did fax the results to our Doctor at the MS clinic. I would then go to a local store and fax the lab paperwork to UT Southwestern. Every month I had to load Sue up and take her to the local Hospital. It didn't matter how hard it was, it seemed worth anything and everything. Then one day we got a call from the MS clinic.

Sue's Doctor Wanda Castro tried her best to see what Sue illness might be. She ran many tests to get a real clear picture of Sue's diagnoses. We were with her for about a year. Dr. Castor was moving to Boston to set up practice in a MS clinic there. The nurse that called said, "She will meet with you two one more time." In this last meeting, we hugged each other and we all cried. It was like losing someone you really needed. We needed her. The last thing I said to her was,

"What is in your gut?"

"What is your gut telling you what Sue has?" I asked.

"In my gut I feel it is Primary Progresses Multiple Sclerosis (PPMS). PPMS is the last stage of MS." She replied.

We left her office in sadness that day. During this time Jennifer was returning on the weekends to visit. She was working two jobs one with the State an hour away and one at a local grocery store. She would stay the night and attempt to help when she could.

"Hey mom, I love you." Jennifer said one afternoon.

Sue smiled brightly.

"I love you too." She said somewhat labored but clear as day.

Jennifer took a step back with notable tears in her eyes yelling at me.

"Hey dad, oh my God! Mom said I love you! I haven't heard her say that in years." Jennifer cried out.

I reached over and gave Sue a kiss on the forehead. No one had heard Sue saying anything especially something as special as those three words in years.

We began to experience problems at the lab though. They were trying to draw blood from her like a normal person. They attempted to un-bend her left arm, which wasn't necessarily an option due to her disease. Her left arm was stiff and unbendable. Sue and I talked to each other in essence shorthand with the laptop. When Sue pecked out a few letters I would know the answer and pick the lap top up and erase it and put it back into her lap for the next word. We were communicating and Sue began to type.

"Take blood out left thumb." The computer said.

"Oh." I said aloud, "I understand now."

I should have known since no one had obtained blood from the bend of the arm in quite some time. I told the lab personnel they needed to take the blood from her left thumb. It went very well, the best drawing of blood in years. I was at work a few days later when Jennifer called. She had better luck then others getting through to me at the prison as she now understood proper procedure having worked for the State now for several months.

"Just to let you know I got a call from APS today. Not really sure what set them off this time. I talked to her for a while though. Let me know if you guys need anything or if I need to talk to them again." She said.

"Alright thanks. Let Travis know I'll be home shortly." I replied.

What could it possibly be now? I thought to myself.

I arrived home and Travis told me that APS had entered the house and were there for two or three hours. We discussed what was going on and how to prepare for another impeding investigation. We knew we weren't doing anything wrong but the stress of an impending investigation on top of everything else was enough to cause any one to boil over. I was extremely frustrated, because APS offered no reasonable help during any of their investigations. Life would have been easier for all of us with just a little more help and a lot less scrutiny.

A couple weeks later, I was at home during my time off. An APS officer came to our home. This APS investigator was a woman who had broken her right hand which was set inside of a cast.

"He is going to write for me," she said as she raised up her casted hand toward my sight.

I noticed that with all of her questions the man was writing feverishly. I thought it was odd but was unsure of why. Finally towards the end of the visit the reason for being investigated was revealed.

"It seems on your last trip to the lab for her testing that you grabbed the laptop in a manner that was described as abuse." She said.

"Oh is that what this is about?" I said slightly confused.

"Some overbearing lab person has just overstepped their bounds. In no way was it even remotely abuse. It's the only way for us to communicate. It was obvious she did not understand how Sue and I communicated."

Once they were finished they began to walk out of the house. The APS worker turned to me as she exited. "Oh," she said, "He is a Highway Patrol Trooper."

By this point I was floored, I felt in some sense tricked. I assumed they automatically thought the worst and brought a law enforcement agent into our house to arrest me should they have seen fit. Yet they did not have the audacity to say anything to me prior to entering my home. Only after everything seemed cohesive did they reveal his true identity. The investigation was closed, and nothing came from it because there was nothing to begin with. In the talks Jennifer had with APS they told her regardless of what claims were made every report or allegation had to be investigated by law to ensure that no abuse whatsoever was taking place.

I thought November 12, 2011 would be a normal day like any other. It was a clear fall day at the prison and everything seemed to be going according to schedule. Yet halfway through my shift I received word of a call waiting for me. I knew by now that no call from anyone to the prison was ever a good sign.

"Dad, it's Jennifer," she said frantically.

"What's going on?" I replied.

"Something happened with Travis. He called me and said he was having hard time breathing because he was bitten by a spider. I told him to call 911 if it was bad but I honestly thought he was overreacting. I couldn't get ahold of him for a second but I finally did and he said an ambulance is on its way."

"Oh God, Ok." I said.

"I'm going to stay at the house until you get home and take care of mom so she's not by herself so don't worry I'll be there." She said.

I knew Jennifer was at least forty five minutes away, but so was I. There was no telling what was even happening at the house while we waited helplessly for word.

When I arrived two and a half hours later Jennifer was sitting in my chair watching TV shows with Sue.

"Ok so what happened?" I asked.

"Well apparently Travis was under the house trying to free a dog and was bitten by a brown recluse or several of them and had an allergic reaction to it. He got back into the house, called me, and thought he was going to be ok. But then he couldn't breathe. He called me back once the ambulance arrived and they asked me how long it was going to take me to get here because they had to leave mom. Took me thirty minutes but I got here. Worst part though they left the door unlocked and her by herself." She said nodding towards Sue.

"God anything could have happened to her," I said.

"Hey be glad I was even up. I had my birthday party last night. So Happy Birthday to me!" Jennifer replied.

Jennifer went to the hospital and sat with Travis while I took care of Sue. It was easier for me to stay at home and prepare for the next day and at least one of us could be there for him. He was maxed out on medicine to combat the reaction and released. I was slightly awake when they finally made it home.

"You ok?" I asked.

"Yeah I just feel bad for mom." Travis replied.

Sue began to wail as Travis tried to console her.

"I'm sorry mom I know that was probably really scary for you to see me on the floor having hard time breathing and not being able to do anything. But I'm ok, it's ok." He said to her as she cried.

We all teared up a little. Sometimes we forgot what it was like for Sue. Yes of course everything was difficult for us but it was unimaginable for her.

In late November 2011 Sue had an infection, and was given the antibiotic Ceftin. I gave this drug to her three times and then noticed that her throat was closing off, almost chocking her to death. I called the Doctor and was told to stop the Ceftin. Sue had suffered another TIA, mini stroke in her brain a few days later.

During this same time I sent an email to everyone I knew just in case they or someone they knew needed to learn what I had learned in caregiving for their families.

Here is the email:

Learn about the illness. In my case I have learned 11 illnesses only to find that any one of them may crop up and have symptoms at any time and last for a few minutes, a few hours, a few days or even months. I have learned to take care of myself. The better I take care of myself the better care I can give care to Sue.

I have learned to set up a business so I can keep on working. I have learned to be on call 24/7. I have learned that Doctors are on call so call them. I have learned that there is never enough money so ask, ask, and ask for help. One can find ways to get help. I have learned to call a RN on my insurance card. Hello RN tells me which way I need to go with this problem. I can call 24 hours a day. I have learned to do things I never thought I ever would do in my life. I have learned to take complete care of my love one for she is totally dependent on someone else to help her do her daily task of living.

I have learned to fight for her. Doctors can care or they can hear from me very loudly. I have learned not to wait. See an infection then do something about it before the infections blows up into something bigger to deal with. I have learned to slow down when I have too. Lord knows I care but there are times I lose all energy and have to go to bed early to get 12 or more hours of sleep.

I have learned not to sweat the small stuff. Get done what you can and to do not worry about the rest. Sometimes the small stuff is not that big of a deal and can be dealt with the next day, next week or not at all. I have learned I do not know it all. God, every day is something else to deal with. I have learned to fight the Insurance Company.

Their first response is always No...So learn that and then ask again. Sometimes there are ways around the No of Insurance Company. I have learned that there are treasurers in care giving. It's not always overwhelming but actually some blessed moments that can be reaped. Look for these moments then go toward that area of life so both caregiver and the one being cared for is blessed. I have learned to give it to God....there are some things that are just not clear....so let go and let God do within His Will and Care.

I have learned I can help others, especially those who are where I was at several years ago. I can be there for them and they can be there for me. I have learned to suck it up. I am not a special care giver. There are others in the same boat as I. Some even worse off than I. I have learned to care...simply be there day in and day out so my love one is blessed. I have learned that others are watching. They are watching from my job, from my church, from my neighbors. All are watching to see how I am handling this ordeal. I have learned and am still learning in my care giving experience.

More experience sure was needed to be learned by me and now I had to learn about how to help Sue with a bed that she choked in every night. Sue was now choking on her own saliva, and I learned she needed extra support that a hospital bed could provide. A friend gave me a hospital bed he no longer needed. The bed did not however, go past thirty degrees wherein the chocking problem laid. I gave the bed away to Hospice once the Insurance said they could get me a rented hospital bed. When I received the rented bed it was the exact same bed I had just gotten rid of. I immediately checked into why these Medicaid approved beds did not go past thirty degrees, and from my research I ascertained someone sued the maker of these beds preventing them from going past thirty degrees. This type of beds would not work for Sue since the beds did not go past thirty degrees. Going past thirty degrees was what was needed to prevent the chocking of Sue each night.

I took Sue to our primary Dr. Tonya Youngblood and told the doctor she chocking on her own saliva.

"She needs a bed that goes forty five degrees to ninety degrees because she's chocking," I said.

The Doctor wrote a prescription that stated,

Need hospital bed that goes 45 to 90 degrees due to aspiration.

I sent the prescription to Hill-Rom bed manufacturer and to our Insurance Company. The Insurance Company was not communicating with me in regards to the issue. Hill-Rom however, told me they were in negotiations. I had just satisfied my deductibles and we were at one hundred percent pay out on insurance needs. I became frustrated as their negotiation continued while Sue kept choking each night. I finally called the Insurance Company.

"I do not know who is negotiating on this Hill-Rom bed, but I know one thing, if my wife dies chocking tonight you can bet I will do an autopsy and if I find she choked on her own saliva then I will sue anyone whose hands are on these negotiations with Hill-Rom." I said exasperated.

The Insurance Company called me the following day telling me that what I had said was not helpful. Yet, they gave Hill-Rom ten days to get this new bed to me. Hill-Rom flew the bed from the State of Indiana into DFW International Airport, and assigned a delivery truck to deliver the bed to my home.

A delivery truck pulled into our cramped driveway containing the hospital bed. I went outside to see if I could assist the driver in getting the bed out of the truck. He opened the sliding door to the back of the truck revealing what looked like a casket.

"This is a hospital bed and not a casket right?" I asked as I turned toward to him.

"Honestly I have no idea." He replied shrugging his shoulders before checking the paperwork.

As I helped the man unload the bed onto the lift and lower the bed to the ground two more vehicles pulled in next to the house. A U-Haul van and what appeared to be a Hill-Rom company truck. Five muscular men and a somewhat scrawny man emerged from the U-Haul van. The six men from the U-Haul began helping us take the bed off of the vehicle lift. Once it was on the ground, the scrawny man began attempting to pull the nailed on wood crated hospital bed apart by his hands only.

"You gotta be kidding me," I thought to myself.

I left for a few moments before returning to the crate with a hammer for the man to use to pry open the box that had been sealed with nails. After removing the nails I peeked into the box and saw it was in fact a hospital bed and not some bizarre miss shipment of a coffin. Once the bed was completely removed from the crate, the delivery driver left leaving me with a lot of men to deal with for one bed.

"You cannot grab the bed by the edges or you will break something." The Hill-Rom resprenstive said to the U-Haul men.

I looked at the bed and then looked back at the doorway. The entry way to our house is extremely narrow, which began to make me feel rather nervous. The hospital bed could not be taken apart and would have to somehow fit through the door. The entire eighteen thousand dollar bed was tied down, leaving nowhere to hold and lift.

The men began scooting the bed slowly while the Hill-Rom representative supervised. I stood from afar not really sure what to do considering seven men were trying to slowly scoot the bed on a concrete pad. Unexpectedly the Hill-Rom representative began taking pictures, followed by one of the men from the U-Haul who also started taking pictures.

"Maybe I better look at this." I said as I walked over to examine the bed,

"Look, I do not care what it looks like when I get it into the home. All I care about is that it works when I get it into the home, so just put the bed inside please."

One of the men finally removed a piano dolly from the van, and an hour later we were able to get the bed up the back ramp and into the house through the back door. Once inside the Hill-Rom representative hooked the mattress into the airlines, and gave me a brief demonstration on how to use the bed. The bed went forty five to ninety degrees, and also produced several different types of modes. A boost mode moved her head down, raised her feet up, making it easier to pull her up in the bed when she slid down too far into the bed. The bed went into chair mode which made it easier to brush her teeth and give her baths. The feet could be extended or shorten as needed. The bed took my back ache away, and was an overall blessing for all of us. The bed had a 911 handle. I pulled it once and Sue got mad at me. I did not know until later after her death when I was in the bed and pulled the 911 handle and the mattress went rock hard. Now I know why Sue got mad at me.

At this point home health nurses were still coming to check in on Sue, and were still helping a few hours a week. *"He's abusive."* Sue typed on the computer to the home healthcare personnel one day.

Normally Sue would receive a bed bath three times a week on Mondays, Wednesdays, and Fridays. On my off days from work I would still give her a regular shower on a shower chair. I began to wash Sue as I often did with a bar of soap. Abruptly Sue began to lose her balance on the shower chair and I attempted to grab her to stop the fall. I was unable to as she literally slipped butt first from the shower chair. I began screaming for help and Travis came and helped me put her back onto the shower chair. Never again did I use bar soap so carelessly. I would soap a part of the body and then rinse it before moving on.

I explained this all to the nurse who had noticed a small bruise on her forearm where I had attempted to grab her to prevent the fall. Regardless of the situation the nurse stated just as the last APS investigator that it would have to be reported and investigated. I braced myself, knowing that yet again I would have to deal with an APS investigation.

Jennifer once again reached me at work letting me know what was going on. As soon as I arrived home from work the APS officer was gone. A couple of days later they came to interview me. Once more there was nothing to it, and the investigation fizzled out into nothing. I know Sue loved me and I knew a lot of her attitude could be attributed to the spots on her brain. The officer stated that Sue relayed that she fell in the shower. I told her of the shower incident and that it was not on purpose but an accident. I got over that investigation, just like the rest and kept going to work. I would tell my supervisors at work to keep them in the loop as added protection as I had done in the past during the other investigations.

February 2012 UT Southwestern called and said they had a supply of Methotrexate. I gladly told them we would be there whenever we needed to be. A week later I went camping again in Sue's hospital room. I took another one hundred dollars and a big suit case in preparation for being at the hospital for at least a week. I knew the nurses loved it when they got the Patterson's. I even heard one of the nurses talking about how I would take care of Sue and they just needed to bring me the items. We had another PICC line inserted again, and the Methotrexate was administered via the IV bag for a second time. They sent us home again with the PICC line, just as they had done the first time. However, the Insurance refused to pay for the treatment a third infusion saying that there were not enough positive results that had come from the treatment itself. Everything was disappointing and shameful about the whole experience. It was a shame that the plant closed as soon as it went Generic. It was a shame that the price was driven up in price due to the shortage of the supply. Our money was in the Insurance and they wanted to keep their money. For the second time in several months I had to yet again request the PICC line be removed by the local hospital as it was of no use to us.

CHAPTER TEN

Thanking God

I had a dental appointment for Sue since she was having problems of a swelling right side of her face. The appointment was on my day off and they canceled it. Of course it was rescheduled for a day I worked, leaving me unable to take Sue. I went to work and Travis took Sue to the dentist. The one time no one was at the house and someone broke into our home. After the back door was kicked in they went on a thrifty burglary spree by stealing all of Sue's Tupperware. Mind you a majority of this Tupperware was from the 80's. Not to mention despite all of the pain medication that was prescribed to Sue, my blood pressure medication was instead stolen.

When Travis arrived at the house he entered through the front door and then returned to the car to start unloading Sue. Travis later relayed to me that he believed the person was still in the house and had most likely hidden behind the kitchen island and grabbed a kitchen knife that was later discovered missing.

When I returned home from work Travis relayed the events of the day, and we called the police to file a police report. He said he waited for me to arrive home so that he could verify what was stolen. After talking to Travis I felt a sense of relief that I had not come home to a double homicide, and that it was only piddle items that were stolen. I took Sue over to her computer on the scooter, pulled up Tupperware online and made an insurance claim for five hundred dollars on the Tupperware. Sue knew that Tupperware is a guaranteed for life product and that we would be able to get full reimbursement for our loss. The back door leaked rain due to them coming into the back door and I was forced to place that on the claim too. We never caught that person which was of great concern to us. If I could have found who broke into my home, they would have hopefully been in jail.

"Talking about kicking a man when he is down, I sure would not want this person or persons as a friend." I told the insurance agent.

Or were they my friends?

I had so many friends before this started with Sue. One by one they left when it became apparent we no longer had anything to talk about. Caregiving had become my life. All I was talking about was the troubles I was going through in caregiving. I thank God for the lady at the doctor office who approached me as I was loading up Sue into the car. "God will bless you for helping her." She said.

I thank God for those at work who would listen to me. I had to get it out of me anywhere I could. I could not hold back what was in me and how I was personally changing. I thank God for my supervisors who supported me and let me take off work each time I needed. I knew if I could find a way to vent then I could keep going. Sue did not ask for her illness, and she was suffering more than anyone could have imagined. We need to respect our love ones and bless them and sacrifice for them. In caregiving that sacrifice is a daily sacrifice.

I was talking to my Attorney Jean about writing a letter to Congress.

"I would do it. In fact I would write it to all of them. You never know who that letter will touch and you might be able to get some help from them as well." She said.

I got to thinking about that one day. I had written a letter to one House member when I just changed the name of each House or Senate member to fit the letter to their office. It took all the night and well into the morning. I got done around 2:30 A.M.

Below is an example of the letter writing campaign, which I sent to one hundred percent of the Senate in Washington D.C and forty five percent of the House of Representatives.

(Look for Letters to House and Senate of the U.S Congressman in the back in Chapter 19.)

I did not know what if anything would come out of this letter writing campaign. I did not expect what did come out of it though. What came out of it was passing the buck and kicking the can down the road. I received email after email after email from North to South and East to West of the United States. I had Senators and House members emailing me for money. That's all I got. No one said I am sorry for your luck. Not one of them cared enough to show me any ways to find funding or help. What was sent to me was already done and flat zero on top of that. I just could not get past the $2,000 rule on any government program. There was no one out there to help us.

And Yet, I still thank God! I thank God for everyone who came into my caregiving world. Those who came in as servants have a special place in my heart now. Those who came into our home to serve us with the mind of Christ, they we not looking for money they were there to serve. Including also where those who helped us in caregiving away from the home, the nurses and Physician Assistance's to the Doctors, Pharmacists behind the scenes who served us away from our home. I thank God for the chance to *do it right* in caregiving. Our story is a story that was done right. You see so many times where things could have and really should have gone wrong and yet God was there each day leading in a special ways. God is so Good to us. I sure do not deserve God's Goodness.

And yet, He freely gives even in caregiving. I could not have done this for Sue without God. I could not have done this without my family. I could not have done this right without everyone who touched my life in special ways. I so needed encouragement and that just what I got. The woman who said God will bless you for helping her. That was really encouraging. The bath women who came into our home, they encourage us. RN and LVN you made your mark on us. Thank God for all of you. Thank God for Hospice and their group. I just cannot express my thanks for you all. I thank God for anyone who came into my world, who listen to me vent, who help me with my needs, who help in many other ways. God I thank You for all who came into our world. It looked so hard and yet You made it so much easier by bringing in the right people in our home to bless us. Thank You God!

CHAPTER ELEVEN

Getting Up Close & Personal

Every six months we would have to change the G-Tube. July 2nd 2012 we were in the bedroom and I was taking off Sue's T-Shirt so I could give her a shower. The G-Tube came completely out of her. I was holding the G-Tube in my hand and a hole was in Sue's stomach. I quickly laid Sue down upon the bed and put pressure on the hole, and placed a pressure bandage dressing on real tight over the whole in her stomach before taking Sue to the hospital immediately. They replaced the G-Tube with a temporary Foley G-Tube and sent us home. Our Doctor was out of state or country at the time and we were forced to wait a week for the stomach wall G-tube to be replaced. The temporary Foley G-tube that went into the stoma was a mess; it did not work as proficiently as the main G-tube did.

When we were first given a G-Tube learning time on how to feed Sue usually caused us complete disarray. The tube was thin and small and would easily become clogged. I learned the easiest way to unclog the tube was to pour Coke into it and let the liquid set for a little while. Coke easily ate away any particles that were left sitting in the tube. The G-Tube contained three valves that opened and at any time if one of the valves opened stomach acid would come through the valve. If a second valve was open and I did not realized it when I would pour 50 ml the Jeivty into the G-tube then 50 ml of Jevity would return through the second opened valve making a mess all over us. Overnight if Sue accidently knocked the valve open I would awaken the next morning to find her and the bed a complete mess. Changing Sue and her bed sheets was an immediate priority that definitely set the mood for the rest of the day.

In early September of 2012 Jennifer was able to make the transition from an Institutional Parole Officer to a District Parole Officer and obtain a position at an office thirty minutes closer to our residence. The only down side was she was required to attend training for five consecutive weeks nine hours away. Her training was slated to begin the first week of October. In hindsight this was the greatest thing she could have ever done.

In October 2012 Travis suffered a serious injury trying to hold Sue as he pulled up her diaper. He damaged the nerve in his left arm, which will most likely affect him for the rest of his lifetime. The Workman's compensation package paid his salary and took care of his medical needs for a few months. Based on his physical injury I was forced to start yet another search for a new employee. Throughout the process ten people said they would take the job only to call me later and decline the job. Some of these people flat out didn't even show for the first day of traning. I requested the entire month of October off which I was granted. I knew Jennifer wouldn't be back until the end of the first week of November to help. I had no idea how I was going to find a new employee. I was grateful to discover that I was making the last payment on our car, which would free up a three hundred and seventy five dollars that was put towards our other bills. At the end of October I decided the best thing for me to do was to go part time at my job. The greatest benefit going part time was the fact that I would only work the weekends. Monday through Friday I became Sue's primary caregiver throughout the week. I now did not have to rely on someone else for the bulk of the caregiving week. The Warden approved me to go part time. Jennifer and I reached an agreement with Travis incapacitated she would come to the house every Saturday and Sunday for at least several hours to help take care of Sue. It prevented her from being able to work both jobs which left her slightly shorthanded every month. I found part time to be mixed blessings.

What I did not know in my part time choice was about to floor me. I knew I would only get one half of my salary. I was making three thousand dollar a month before taxes and brought home around twenty four hundred dollars after all the deductions were taken out. What I did not know was that I had to pay half of my Insurance premium and all the premiums for Sue's Insurance, which meant I was paying around eight hundred dollars a month just for Insurance premiums in part time work. I brought home after deductions five hundred and thirty three dollars a month. That was a big hit to take all of a sudden in our budget. That was an eighteen hundred and sixty seven dollar hit each month. The blessings in part time work did allowed me to be able to devote almost all of my time directly to the care of my sweetheart. Monday through Friday and 5 P.M to 10 P.M on the weekends I took care of her. I was slated to begin working part time on December 9th 2012.

It was just not a financial hit I took when I went part time. It was also a physical hit. I knew going into part time that I was going to be in a world of hurt. Weekends at a prison entail visitation which means standing and possible patting down (or as we call it shaking down) visiting person's at the prison for ten hours on each of those two days. I knew by the time I would finish with Sue over the course of those five days that I would be physically and emotionally exhausted. There would be no room for recovery between my days off and my work days.

I took Sue back to the MS clinic at UT Southwestern.

"She is long term," said the Doctor.

"I knew that some 2 years ago." I replied.

The Doctor had another person to come into the room to sit with Sue while he pulled me into another room. We went into another office where another woman was setting awaiting for us to enter the office. The doctor turned to me and said,

"What's going to happen if you get hurt?"

"I am screwed if that happens." I replied.

"That's no plan!!" He said as he jumped up reaching for a pamphlet for a Lawyer.

"You will have to cover the first two months of a Nursing home and these lawyers will get Sue Medicaid to pay for her stay from then on." The Doctor said handing me a pamphlet.

"I do not want to do that. In fact I don't even have the money to do that for two months." I said to him.

That evening I devised a plan and emailed it to the Doctor. I told him as of that point we were practically living on her income. If I got hurt, I would have her income to pay for someone to come into our home and take care of both of us. I could quit my job and get my retirement and pay monthly bills for eighteen months and then go back and get my job back. The option was readily available to me due to the shortage of staff statewide. After sending this email to the doctor I feared a safe run by him through our house.

I looked around the house which was really in despair. My dish washer had not worked for the last four years. The stove top leaned from side to side. The deep freezer top was so broken that it was cooling my home. And I was so tired; I really needed some type of comfortable chair. My recliner broke down years ago. The recliner was in fact the only piece of "living room" furniture we had owned in years because the hospital bed took up so much space. I made the decision go to the web for Conn's Home Plus. I did "Yes Money" credit application. They gave me six thousand dollars in credit. I did not need six thousand dollars but I did spend around fifteen hundred dollars. I needed to make some upgrades around the house. I did not want a doctor to do a safe run in the current condition of my house. If for nothing else, I bought these things for my own sanity. I bought a new dishwasher, a new stove with a glass top and a new stand up freezer. I additionally labeled exits and stuck 911 packs onto the walls again.

I found out that, I was passionate about Sue's care. Maybe too passionate for my own good, she slowly began to lose her ability to use her hands and fingers. Once that ability was gone she was no longer able to communicate on her laptop. Since she could not speak words either, it did not take an hour of her whining before I went running to Office Depot. I mean I took off fast in the car and got to that store. I told them our situation and he showed me the aisle I was in dire need of. I bought an easel, a board and dry erase markers. I had seen on a TV show *"Breaking Bad"* a situation almost identical to ours.

There was a scene where an old man was in a Nursing home and could not speak. He had a bell on his wheel chair, and the nurse had an alphabet board. When she passed the vertical numerical row that contained the number the man wanted he would ring the bell. The nurse would then horizontally proceed down that row and upon passing the letter he wanted he would again ring the bell. The nurse would spell the word out as she went revealing what the man was trying to say. I started watching reruns of *Breaking Bad* in an attempt to find this one scene I was searching for. I watched a few shows but could not find the scene of the old man in the nursing home. I Google alphabet boards and found one like they had on the show.

Here is how we communicated:

The BOARD:

1	2	3	4	5	6
A	B	C	D	M	N
E	F	G	H	S	T
I	J	K	L	Y	Z
O	P	Q	R		
U	V	W	X		

As I would go across the numbers Sue would blink, move her head, or lift her first finger when I got to the row. As I went down the rows in order to find the correct letter she would again stop me one of those ways. We spelled out words in order to communicate with each other. It was quite the pain in the butt and was quite the blessing at the same time. It sometimes took a lot of time to find and spell out the correct words.

For example, I would ask Sue what number it was? 1, and she blinked her eyes. Ok row one what letter is it? A, E I; she blink on I. Ok so I what? Is I the subject and she blinked. Ok I space. Row 1, 2, 3, 4 she blinked, ok what letter is it? D, H, L; she blinked on L. Ok I L what? Row 1 and she blinked. Ok letter A, E I, O; she blinked on O. Ok I LO. Row 1, 2; she blinked on 2. Ok letter B, F, J, P, V; she blinked on V. Ok I Lov is it Love I asked. And she nodded Yes. Ok; I love what? 1, 2, 3, 4, 5 she blinked on 5. Letter M, S, Y; she blinked on Y. I love Y. I think I know but let's make sure. Row 1 she blinked on 1. So letter A, E, I, O; she blinked on O. Ok I know what you are saying. Is it: I Love You. She nodded her head forward yes and I was blessed to know that Sue can self-express herself and be heard now.

Later I made a YouTube video on this communication board. If you would go to YouTube site and type into the search bar: *How to communicate with your loved one when they lose the ability to speak* and you will find this video to help you communicate with your love one when they no longer can speak or type out words on a computer.

Jennifer left in October for her scheduled training and we were all sad to see her go.

"*Surely*," I thought to myself, "*As long as everything goes right this next month we will be in good shape.*"

Nothing went right; in fact it all went terribly wrong.

CHAPTER TWELVE

Sad Days

Near the end October 2012 Jennifer called me to say that Sue's younger sister was found dead in her home. Due to Sue's illness it would be impossible for us to travel to the funeral in Missouri to pay our respects. I took my time telling Sue trying to find the right moment to break this sad news to her.

"I have to tell you something very sad. Your sister Shannon has been found dead in her home." I said.

Telling Sue was not easy and she immediately became upset and flooded with emotion. It was a very difficult few days for us. It was tough to tell her, it was tough to receive but I held Sue in my arms and prayed with her. The next several days were trite with emotion for both Sue and I.

November 8th, 2012 was starting out as a typically exhausting day. It was the day of Sue's sister's memorial and I knew it was important to try and keep Sue's mind off of it. My day's usually started around 3 A.M. and once my feet hit the floor Sue's daily schedule would start. I was feeding Sue through her G-Tube when my phone began to ring. I could not reach the phone while holding the syringe and pouring the Jeivty into her body. Multitasking was not an option while G-Tube feeding.

Once I grabbed the phone I saw an email from Travis titled, *it is finished*. I pondered to myself what that possibly meant when I saw the missed calls were from Jennifer who was still nine hours away in Beeville, Texas doing the training for her job. The training was based on exams that the employee was required to pass. On this particular day she was supposed to take her final, should she fail the final she would be fired.

"Hello." I said.

"Dad you need to go back to Travis' bedroom. I got a bunch of texts from him and he's trying to commit suicide right now." She said frantically.

"What are you talking about?" I replied.

I did not have my hearing aids in and had caught only bits and pieces of what she said.

"Dad I called the police and have been trying to get a hold of you for the last few minutes. An ambulance and police are on their way. Travis is trying to kill himself go to the room." She panted.

That time I heard it, I heard her saying her brother was attempting suicide. I ran to the back bedroom and as I neared it I heard loud music. I pushed open the door and turned the light on. Lying around him in his bed were pictures of three of his children. At this point in time he was non responsive. I suddenly heard a loud knock right as police kicked the door open to our home. I hung the phone up on Jennifer who was still listening.

I hurried back to Sue who was left propped up in her scooter at the table. I knew I needed to be out of the way for the emergency personnel and I knew that Sue was sitting helpless as she watched the police and paramedics storm our house. We discovered that Travis had consumed an entire bottle of Tylenol, he was rushed to the local hospital where is stomach was pumped and he was put under suicide watch.

Jennifer and I were in communication throughout the whole day. She took the final for her job, and passed. The administrators were gracious enough to allow her to leave a day early so that she could at least go sit with Travis. It was the day before her birthday and she was busy speeding from Beeville to our home to make sure everything was ok. Jennifer went and visited Travis and so did I when I could get away. The hospital was keeping him and then transferring him to a mental health hospital in Dallas.

Death was rushing into our home while Sue sat there to witness it, feel it and not be able to do anything but accept it. It was a messy time and we continued on our work with Sue's caring for her daily needs. Despite all of the emotions we were feeling we could not just simply stop. Sue still had to be cared for and we were doing our best to move forward.

CHAPTER THIRTEEN

Harder Days

One day I look at Sue and found her in a puzzling way. For four hours she looked just like a shell of a person. It looked like nothing was going on upstairs. I had explained this to her Doctors. They did not say much about that but it left me wondering. In February it snowed eight inches of snow. In Texas, that is a huge problem. The roads get a mess and cars going flying all over the place off the slick road. Sue started throwing up a green substance. I called the twenty four seven Nurse Line with the Insurance company. They told me to get her to the hospital. In the snow we went to the Hospital. The doctor said that it was probably something she ate that did not agree with her. I know all she gets is Jeivty and throwing up green bile is not good!

Every year I have a hard week in my job called In-Service. It is long days filled with exercise, gun shooting and testing. Normally I wouldn't consider it to be so draining but I was exhausted from taking care of Sue. Failure to any part during In-Service were met with severe consequences which could ultimately lead to being fired.

Travis was recently transferred from the nicer private mental health hospital he was staying at for approximately a week to the State mental hospital. He had been there for several weeks and showed no sign of being released. Jennifer was also forced to take off work during my In-Service training to care for Sue. No one else was available and In-Service was required for every Correctional Officer and all Non-Uniform employees each year. I was at the point that I was so tired I could not even take care of myself.

Travis wasn't released until the end of November after Thanksgiving. We took turns visiting him since one person had to stay behind to care for Sue. When he came home he was different. He was given a diagnosis for a mental health condition and ordered to take mountains of pills or he would be forcibly taken back to the State hospital. He still attempted to help with Sue's care to the best of his ability.

I noticed in the beginning of December what appeared to be a hole no larger than a pen point on Sue's bottom. I turned to researching bed sores on the internet thinking it was the only logical conclusion. I looked at the steps that were written on how to treat the sore which included cleaning the sore, giving air to the sore and turning every two hours to keep pressure off the sore.

"You know that little fan truckers use in their cabs?" I asked Travis because he once was a truck driver.

"You can get that at Walmart." He replied.

I went to town and bought a clip on fan. I would turn Sue on her side; clip on that fan to the bed and blow air onto her sore then turn her every two hours. I would ask Sue if she wanted to watch TV or listen to music. The music allowed for the hospital bed to stay in its exact location however, when she wanted to watch a movie it required unplugging the bed and turning it so the bed was facing the TV directly. We all did our hardest to have her turned every two hours for twelve hours out of the day. She was turned so much that she stopped lying on her left side. The sore went from a pencil head to a dime, to a nickel to a quarter to a half dollar size in no time.

The Hospice RN Vicky told me,

"I know you are doing all that you can. It might mean that she is dying. Sores that will not heal are part of the dying process."

I could lay Sue's hospital bed to the angle of my recliner. It felt and looked like when we were in bed together like we had been for all those years. Sue used to drive me crazy when we were in bed together. She wanted to talk and I wanted to sleep, but I missed those days like none other now.

Once I brought her into this position, while I sat in my chair, I would look into her eyes and told her, "You are so beautiful to me." She started to cry and a tear rolled down her face.

I would gently wipe her tears away with a Puff.

"That's what you are. Just beautiful to me, I love you so much," I said to her.

"I am a better man because of you."

"I love you so much Sue, I going to miss you!"

"I treasured you and will always treasure you."

We would sometimes lie like that and put on music. She loved the 70's station on the satellite called Sonic. We turned out the lights, put the channel on Sonic and would rest together. It was nice because we both needed rest. These days were very beautiful. They became precious memories to me now and quite sweet to remember them now.

In March 2012, I was sick, with the flu. I had to stay as far away from Sue as possible. The last thing I wanted was for her to catch it. I feared Sue catching not just the flu but even the common cold. It would have been very detrimental to her since she has such a comprised immune system. I called Jennifer immediately and begged her to come to the house to help with Sue. She took several days off and came to the house to do what she could with Sue. It caused a rift with her and her immediate supervisor, which later led Jennifer to the decision of transferring to a different office.

The flu kicked my behind. When I got up nine days later, I made sure I no longer had fever and went back to caring for Sue. I thank God for Jennifer and Travis they had been such a great help in these awful days of caregiving.

On April 19ᵗʰ, 2013 at 1 P. M, I called Hospice.

"It is time for my wife Sue Patterson to be placed into Hospice." I said.

They were at my house an hour later doing the intake into Hospice. Comfort drugs came to my door some one hundred and twenty miles away that were driven right to my door. We started the process of *Palliative Care*. I had resolved that Sue due to the shortage of chemo would not get better. By bringing Hospice into the home; we went from *Curative Care* to *Palliative Care*. *Palliative Care* is not Curing but Comforting.

When I called Hospice I was still giving Sue showers in the shower.

"What wrong her toe nails?" I asked Vicky.

They looked black and some were falling off. For weeks I asked the RN what does this mean. Then one day, I was pulling Sue out of the shower when I noticed that her toe was bleeding. I sat her into the scooter and put pressure on her toe. One of the toe nails was barely hanging on. Then I figured out what was going on with her toes. I did not know it, but I was having a hard time lifting her out of the shower now. I put Sue in the hospital bed and called Hospice.

"I want bed baths from now on five days a week. I will no longer be giving Sue showers because I do not have the strength anymore to clear the shower door track and I am ripping her toe nails off." I said.

From that day on I no longer was doing showers. Hospice sent a full time bed bath lady in. We did not like the way she was giving baths. After a few baths, Sue told me on the board to fire her. I called Hospice and ask for someone else to be sent for the bed baths. They sent us another woman who Sue absolutely adored named Brenda. She did a great job of cleaning Sue in the bed. You could tell she cared as she gave the bath. I would assist Brenda with Sue's bath by lifting her legs so Brenda could clean around her legs and then I would put Aquaphor, grease like substance, on Sue's feet so pressures sores would not develop on her feet. I would lay Sue on her side and hold her so Brenda could clean her backside and personal area.

Brenda was faithful and she did a great job. We had fun all three of us as we bathed Sue. We had laughs and told stories, sharing our lives as we served Sue. Sue had a way to get you laughing rolling all over the floor. Sue was a real blessing at times to serve her. I will never forget when she had me spell out on the board,

"Thank You for helping me."

That ripped my heart out. She had never said that before, and yet it made all of our hardships worth it.

August 14, 2013 as soon as I fed Sue the two shakes with water, Sue went into convulsions, I opened back up her G-Tube and drained out 500 ml of the 1,000 ml of Jeivty and water. I called Hospice and three nurses came rushing out to my home. Brenda was in the house administering Sue's bath when it occurred. I told Brenda to grab a brown bag that was on top the counter. I folded the brown bag and put it over Sue's mouth. She calmed down a little after that, I had enough.

I thought about killing myself. I said, NO to suicide though and went on with what I was doing. I was going to town to sign Sue up for a State I.D card since she could not renew her license anymore. I was standing in line waiting at The Texas Department of Motor Vehicle, (TxDMV) when I made the decision to make myself an organ donor. My thoughts and ideologies had completely changed since I started caregiving. Once I signed Sue up for home visit they called me to see when they could come out and take her picture. A week later I received her ID card in the mail.

The next day I had a Hospice person in the room. Sue had me spell out on the board,

"He is mean to me."

Later the Social worker came over and she spelled out to her the same message. I was in my car a few days later when my cell phone rang. On the other end of the line was this Hospice Social Worker.

"John I know you keep your home clean and I know you are taking very good care of Sue. I know if Sue was put into a home she would quickly decline. But I am bound by law; I have to turn you into APS. I am sorry." She said.

The APS officer came into my home a week or so later.

"You have history!" She said.

"The only history I had," I thought, *"Was being accused of frivolous things."*

Sue had me spell out on the board, *"John needs counseling."*

The APS officer and I went to the porch.

"The charge was verbal abuse and hitting." She said.

"No way!" I replied.

We stood out there for a good while turning the conversation over to what was going on in our State jobs. A few weeks later the APS worker returned to our house.

"We found someone to come into the home and give you both counseling. Sue will also need to go into Nursing home every six weeks as Respite care for your benefit John," she said.

I cringed at both thoughts. Doing counseling together would be impossible with that board. It would take an hour just to spell out anything Sue wanted to say in just a few words. And putting her into a Nursing home, for Respite Care was out of the question. Again I was left feeling there was no plausible help. All I needed was a few extra hands coming into my house to help with Sue and I couldn't even be given that.

I saw a spider one day by my desk. Between Sue's inability to defend herself from any type of bug and Travis' terrible allergic reactions I knew we needed to spray the house. I arranged for Sue to be placed into Respite Care at a Nursing home for seventy two hours. In seventy two hours I could bomb the house for insects and clean my kitchen floor.

I went to the nursing home to look over the area. A woman there showed me a room with a bed much like what we had at home. When I got Sue there though that day, she was in a semi-private room in an old Medicaid approved bed that did not go past thirty degrees. I got Sue settled and showed the nurse a smaller maker board so Sue could communicate with them.

"Where is the TV?" I asked the nurse.

"We will get one in here." She replied.

I went home and spent hours on my knees, cleaning the kitchen floor with a bottle of ammonia. Jennifer was there to help me while I cleaned the house from top to bottom. After the kitchen was finished Jennifer and I went to visit Sue. We checked in on her at 5 P.M. Jennifer arrived first and told me when she entered the room she saw five women crowded over Sue trying to figure out what she wanted. Once the room cleared Sue spelt out for Jennifer the following.

"I did not get my shake. And they told me to poop in my diaper."

When I arrived at the room it was hot. It felt ninety degrees and Sue's illness reacted poorly to heat. I paid the price throughout Sue's care to have the home at seventy degrees year round. That was very costly but it was more costly to let Sue get hot. Sue's illness did so poorly in heat. Jennifer quickly pulled me to the side to tell me what had happened. I immediately headed for the Nurses' station.

"I want the person who is taking care of Mrs. Patterson and someone in Authority to be in her room in five minutes." I said.

They both came into Sue' room,

"Why has she not been feed lunch? Its supper time and she's not had lunch. What's wrong with this picture?" I asked.

The male nurse started feeding Sue's supper through the G-Tube.

The Authority person told me she would call the nurse who was there at lunch. She left the room with the cell phone to her ear. The person in Authority came back into the room.

"She said a patient had fallen and she just forgot about your wife." She said.

"That's no excuse. There's no excuse for not feeding her lunch. She cannot feed herself!" I exclaimed.

Jennifer figured out it was six hours since Sue's last meal. I was beyond mad, I was livid. I additionally demanded to know why the room was so hot.

"I wanted a sign on that door to keep the door closed to keep the room cooled off." I told the nurse. I kissed Sue and went home; I was just too tired and exhausted from the day. I was so tired and worried though I could not sleep.

I called RN Vicky and told her several things I wanted Hospice to order for the nursing home to follow. Travis was up so we bug bombed the house and went to town. We killed some time overnight at Walmart and we went to I-Hop to eat. We bombed inside the house, under the house and sprayed the yard. I got the house aired out and instead of seventy two hours, I went and pulled Sue out of that nursing home. I thought in forty eight hours she would have been dead the way they were treating her. We had to wait ten days before we could clean up the house. I was not going to have any spiders or any other insects crawling on Sue.

The day came where another hard decision had to be made. When would we do the last paper work: The Living Will? Sue was getting bad, and she was down to only a working mind. We had been communicated better by this time I had gotten pretty good with the communication board. I had done the board so much I had it memorized. I took my cell phone and acted like I was going to send a text and went over to the recliner and talked to Sue.

Sue would still stop me when I got to the numbers or letters and I would put that letter in text form. The text would give "suggestive words," allowing me to guess much faster what she was trying to say. I told Sue we had to talk about the end.

"I hate to and I know you hate to as well but we need to decided so I can do what you want me to do for you." I said.

We agreed on October 2013 to start the Living Will. That date was picked due to Sue having one last prescription that would run out on that date. She always demanded that I get that prescription filled and put it in her shake. Suddenly during these times, I found some ways to meet our financial needs.

I found out that some Life Insurance companies had a rider built into their policies called *Accelerated Death Benefit*. I got the $5000 pretty fast through my job. The money went quick. I did not realize just how much we as a family were doing without. I cashed in another Insurance policy for $10,000. I did another *Accelerated death benefit* with AAA Life Insurance Company. They would only release one-half of the money and then took out another $400 for services. I kept $4,000 in the bank. I will use that for the transformation back to full time at work. I will have to work a month in order to start getting paid again.

CHAPTER FOURTEEN

The End of Caregiving: The Living Will

Day 1, On August 22, 2013 at 10 A.M., I was in my recliner watching TV with Sue. It was not unusual for me to lay in the recliner and put on whatever station Sue wanted to watch. Most days the TV would play on while we both napped. She moaned like she wanted to say something so I grabbed my cell phone. She communicated to me and said,

"What good is a Living Will if you are not going to ever start it?"

"Honey we both agreed on October." I replied.

I looked into her eyes.

"Do you really want to start The Living Will today?" I asked her.

"Yes." She motions her head.

I got mad, I mean really mad! I did not want to starve Sue. The purpose of the Living Will was so Sue could state on her own terms when she wanted lifesaving efforts abolished which included withholding of food and water.

"Do you really want to start the Living Will?" I asked again.

Again she nodded, yes.

"Are you sure this is what you want now?" I asked. Sue again nodded her head yes.

I went over to the stack of Jeivty and threw all of it into the trash can. I picked up my phone and called Hospice. I had been warning them for weeks that she was leaning toward the Living

Will. I told Hospice that Sue wanted to start her Living Will today. I called an Attorney that dealt with *End of Life* decisions, and faxed a copy of her Living Will to this attorney. The attorney relayed to me that I was covered and we could proceed on with the Living Will. RN Vicky came to our house and reassured me that it was Sue's right to make the decision and I was doing right by her. Vicky told me Sue would continue to survive for ten to twelve days and that she would probably just stop breathing.

Sue and I knew that this was going to be the end of her life on this earth. She sure had more guts than I did. I did not want to lose her but I did not want to see her in the continued pain she was in either. I became confused, and in some ways felt as though I was in shock. I hated the fact that the only way to grant Sue's wishes were to take away food and water, and that there was not another option for her. During this time frame for every person who entered the house that was associated with Hospice I would ask Sue if she wanted to stop the Living Will, each time Sue would spell out on the board she wanted to continue the Living Will.

Day 4, Hospice brought in a new Social Worker who came into our home on the fourth day.

"Sue do you want to stop the Living Will?" I asked heading to the board to await her response.

"*No.*" She replied while shaking her head.

"Sue would you like counseling while we are doing this?" The social worker asked.

"*No.*"

Later in the day I received a call from a previous APS officer who had been involved with us.

"I hear Sue has decided on a life ending decisions." The officer stated.

"Yes I am sorry to say she has." I replied.

"Well if you ever need anything please feel free to call us."

I thanked the officer and hung up the phone.

Day 5, Hospice sent a physician assistant into my home. She performed an assessment of Sue and turned to me.

"You have taken great care of her." She said.

She was looking at her feet, peering down at the stuffed dog toy between her feet.

"That's how we have kept her feet from crossing over one another into restrictions." I said.

She high fived me, telling me I had done a great job again.

"Let me see the Living Will please." She said.

I went over to my filing area and grabbed the Living Will out of my book. The PA read over the documents before turning back to me.

"I see this was done in 2009. Was she in sound mind when she signed?" She asked.

"Yes," I replied.

Day 6, Sue was still having great pain everyday so I called Hospice who sent the older PA to our house. Sue stated her pain level was at a 10. The PA put an order into the pharmacy for Methadone as she explained it was the last resort to controlling pain. The pain patch was applied to Sue's skin and required being replaced every seventy two hours and I was told to give Sue the Methadone three times per day as well. Vicky questioned that decision, and so did I but I knew the PA had more education then us so surely she knew what she was doing. Two days of that combination and Sue passed out. She went into a drug induced coma. On Monday Vicky called the Pharmacy, and explained to them the order that was in place.

"That is way too much! Stop the Methadone and the pain patch. They are both long term drugs in the body," said the pharmacist.

"How long will it take Methadone to get out of her body?" I asked.

"Nine days," he replied.

When Sue recovered from the pain medication overdose she talked about how hard this was. I told her, "It was hard for all of us."

"Do you want to stop this Living Will?" I asked again.

"*No*," was her reply on the board.

Brenda and I changed out Sue's catheter due to blockage in tube. We all knew the end of her may be near.

On Day 8, Sue said she was hungry, and had an emotional breakdown.

"Do you want to stop this Living Will?" I asked.

"*No*." Was her reply on the board?

I told Sue she could have some Mt Dew and I went to the freezer and got a couple spoonful of ice cream and went over to Sue and feed her a little bit, just enough to take the edge off of her hunger.

Neither I nor anyone else in the family cooked during the Living Will. None of us wanted Sue to endure the smell of food throughout the house. I vividly remember going to the laundry room and eating in solidarity just to be away from Sue so she would not see me eating. We mostly had stuff to make sandwiches and snack style things to eat.

On Day 9, I asked her if she wanted Mt Dew. I notice instead of the normal aspiration when she consumed the drink, she drank it normally. Then I noticed that her tensed up body had gone limp, and her right bent arm was loosening. There was too much space between her feet; she no longer needed the stuffed dog anymore. I sat in my recliner and Sue was on her right side. I looked into her eyes and said,

"If they pray in Heaven then pray for me. I am going to be really lonely without you. I love you so much. You made me a better man. I love you Sue, I will always love you. I need you so much."

Tears rolled down our cheeks as she nodded.

On Day 10, Sue's sisters came down from Missouri. Her sister Mary is a former RN, and her younger sister Yvonne currently works for a nursing home. Mary took all of Sue's comfort drugs and created a coherent schedule. Her sister's stayed for couple of days and tried to help where they could before returning to Missouri. This schedule put Sue into another drug induced coma. I stopped the schedule that Mary had made up. When Sue awoke she had the most beautiful smile, wide smile, on her face and she was looking up toward Heaven. It was the most beautiful look I have ever seen on anyone's face before.

On Day 12, Sue asked me how long she would live. Sue at this point had surpassed the date that the Doctors thought she would live without food or water. I told Sue she was in the ball park on first base. Sue was well hydrated throughout her care, after all I gave her approximately six gallons of water per month. I wondered if this was perhaps why she was surviving longer than anticipated.

On Day 13, Sue took a bad turn that night. I thought it would take seventy two hours or less for her to pass away. She was still putting out to much urine and was considered to be extremely hydrated. I told Sue she was on second base.

On Day 14, Brenda came in and gave a bed bath to Sue. Brenda would not say goodbye to her knowing that this was the last time she would come to our home and give Sue a bath.

I held it together in front of her, but when I got out to the car I lost it, she would later text to me.

Jennifer, Travis and I had devised a specific schedule for watching Sue. I was taking care of her during the day, and Jennifer would take over around 7 P.M. At around 1 A.M. Travis would take over and tend to Sue until I was up and ready to take care of her again at 3 A.M. Before going to bed I told Sue I thought she was on third base.

On day 19, I woke at 4 A.M. and lay in bed for around thirty minutes. I did not want to get up for some reason. Jennifer burst into the room unexpectedly.

"Mom's breathing is not good," she said. "She's stopped breathing several times in the night and started again but I think she's about to pass."

I got out of bed and put on fresh clothes while Jennifer tried to wake Travis. I took one look at Sue and was taken back by how she reminded me of a character straight out of a zombie movie. Her mouth was going up and down in a relaxed motion. She would stop breathing and then start up again.

"She is gasping, gasping is not breathing," I thought to myself.

I told Jennifer to grab our stethoscope and place it upon her chest.

"Start counting her heart beats when I tell you." I said.

I waited for the 2nd hand on the clock to reach the 12.

"Go." I said.

30 seconds later.

"Stop," I said. "How many did you count?"

"50" Jennifer replied.

50 I thought, times 2 = 100 beats per minute.

"She is still alive and she is still trying so hard to breathe."

I took Sue' oxygen line off, and brought her head up in the bed by raising her upper body up in the bed.

"Honey run for home plate, run for Heaven," I whispered into her ear.

I went into prayer whispering into Sue's ear for God to take her at that moment.

Jennifer later said she heard the last breathe. And when she heard her last breath Sue smiled widely before letting go. I laid Sue back down flat on the bed. I pulled the sheet up to her head. Only her face was showing.

I called Hospice immediately at 5:00 A.M., shortly after her passing. I told Hospice I believed my wife had just passed away. They informed me the RN lived in the same town as me, and he would be there within minutes. The minutes seemed like hours but, the RN was at our house by 5:20 A.M. He looked into her eyes, and listened for a breath.

"Are you calling her dead at this time?" I asked.

"Yes." He said.

At 5:28 A.M. on September 7th 2013 Sue was pronounced dead. Once the RN pronounced Sue has passed, I pulled the sheet over her head. The Hospice RN called the Will Body Program at UT Southwestern, and they asked the RN numerous questions to make sure her body was still a Candidate for the program. Once he was off the phone he turned to me.

"They will be here in a couple of hours to pick up the body." He said.

While we were waiting he started taking care of the various other duties he had to do.

"Where are her narcotics?" He asked.

I showed him where they all were lined up in a row.

"Do you have coffee grounds, kitty litter or tea bags?" He asked.

We searched the cabinets and found tea bags.

"That will work; grab three of the tea bags." He said.

He opened the tea bag and put them in a quart Zip Lock bag. He poured all the drugs into the bag by taking all the drugs out of their capsules, mixing them all up together. He went over to the sink added water and shook up the bag before throwing it into the trash. I signed off with him time and date of when we had destroyed all her drugs.

I received a call from UT Southwestern that they were having trouble finding the house. I directed them into my driveway. They exited their Hurst and wheeled a gurney up our ramp through the back door. Once they reached Sue's body they stopped.

"Can we wrap her up in these fitted sheets?" One of the women asked.

"Yes you can." I replied.

They pulled the fitted sheets off the hospital bed and slipped it over Sue's body. Once I put the sheet over Sue's head at 5:28 A.M. I did not see her body ever again. They took her body away. I had been grieving for years or so I thought. I lost it once her body was wheeled away, I cried all day. The next day Travis and I went to church. We had to wait until Monday before we could finalize all of the arrangements for Sue's memorial. It was a long weekend, and time felt as though it had slowed so very down. Every hour felt as though it was lasting for six hours.

On Monday Jennifer and I went to the Funeral Home. We picked out the book for people to sign, flowers and various other memorial related items. We decided on that Saturday a week later to have the memorial for Sue, allowing Sue's family enough time to arrange a trip from Missouri. Included in the memorial was a CD featuring pictures of Sue with Butterflies floating around, as well as music to accompany it. Songs included in the CD were "*You are so Beautiful*" by Joe Crocker, "*I will Always love you*" by Whitney Houston, and "*In the Arms of an Angel*" by Sara McLachlan. The Pastor and the Song Leader of our church also sung, Sue's favorite Hymn, "The Old Rugged Cross."

The Pastor during his sermon made a beautiful gesture. He said if Sue can blink with her eyes, and use to board in an effort to talk about Jesus we should use our speech to witness about Jesus.

Here is a poem that Sue wrote in 2004:

Jesus

Jesus, King of kings, Lord of lords,
Satan trembles at Your Name. Since I've
Found You, I'll never be the same.
Saved, saved, and saved. Let us shout it
From the roof tops, let us sing it in our
Schools. Saved and I don't care who
Knows
It, or that I'm breaking any rules.
Forgive me where I fail you, increase
My Faith each day. I know there's more

Work on Earth to be done, so I'll carry
On. I'm so glad God sent You, His one and
Only son
Saved, saved, saved. Let us shout if
from the roof tops, let us sing it in our
schools. Saved and I don't care who
Knows
It, or that I'm breaking any rules.
Help us to grow in Faith and do God's
Perfect Will. Let us give thanks in
Everything. Bring Joy and Happiness as
We Praise Your Name.
Sue Ann Patterson, Copyright 2004

The next day after Sue's memorial Jennifer and I chose two plants we wanted to keep. I took the remainder of the beautiful memorial flowers to two nursing homes. I knocked upon their doors and offered the flowers for their patients. I saw smiles on all the faces as they showed me where to put the beautiful flowers. They were blessed and I was blessed for not throwing out the flowers but giving the flowers to those who needed them the most after Sue's memorial.

After the memorial service for Sue, I took day three, day five and day seven and I dumped this book out into a file on the computer. I had to get it out of me, I could not take it anymore and I felt as though this was a way to help me in my Grief. Caring for Sue had taken so much out of me the last six years and six months. (By the way, that was the worst thing I could have done for this book. I was so messed up and wow did it show in the book. The book was fragmented like my life was. In pieces some things here and other things strung over there. I was really messed up and so was the book. It took two years of re-writing the book. The re-writes piled up to 24 inches in height.)

That Friday, There was a knock at the door of our home. The person at the door was handing out letters that they had a break in a main water line and that the water was going to be shut off for the duration of the weekend. I had planned that weekend to go to a Methodist church in Frisco, Texas to thank them for helping us out in our care giving experience.

"Let's go on vacation and go to Frisco and then we will not have to get up early and go on Sunday." Travis said.

"Alright let's do it." I replied.

We both packed a bag and took off for Frisco, Texas. I had just bought a GPS system and this was a good time to try it out on the road.

The Serenity Church in the Colony, Texas was the church that prayed us through hard nineteen days of the Living Will. These were hard days and it sure was a blessing to know that during that time Souls from all over the world were praying for Sue and I. We went to Serenity Church and I asked the Pastor If I could thank them for helping us in care giving. The Pastor let me step up to the mike and I thank them. After the service a young man came to me.

"You do not recognize me do you?" He said.

"No sir I do not, why?" I asked.

"You were the officer that scared me straight when I was a child. I had gotten into so much trouble that the Judge said the scared straight program was my last chance." He replied.

It took a second but I remembered the boy. I had locked up both top and bottom cells and told the inmates of the county jail to scare the wits out of this kid that was about to come into the dorm. I told the inmates to bang the heck out of the doors knowing that when they did the sound bounces off the walls and quickly sinks into ones Soul. The kid came in and I set him down on one of the day room tables.

"How would you like to live here?" I asked.

Wow! Did the inmates raise heck in that moment, it was like a riot. It felt like such a great blessing, to know I had helped this young person so many years ago. It brought me joy during this bleak time in my life.

Twenty days after Sue's passing, three men came from Waco, Texas. They had come to interview me about Real Time praying on www.Guidepost.org.

They asked me many questions about Real Time praying. I told them I prayed all over the world, and that it was a global ministry. They held a men's prayer group in the church they attend in Waco. I told them, it is one thing to be in a single prayer group in your home church, it's another thing to pray globally. People click on that button for prayer from faraway places. People who are suicidal click on for prayer. People from many Faiths click on, you will have to treat each person the same and pray on. Praying on is what I must do in my life.

I called UT Southwestern daily after ten days looking for a Death Certificate. Each time I would press two for Death Certificates and leave my name and number. Each time no one called. Then one day, instead of pressing two I accidentally pressed eight on the phone. The phone started to ring so I let the phone ring and a live person answered the phone.

"Hello, how may I help you today?" She said.

"Yes this is John Patterson and I looking for a Death Certificate on my wife Sue Patterson. I am about to go into Probate and need that Death Certificate." I said.

"Hang on I am going to transfer you over to another person who can help you better," she said.

Another person answered and I explained to her what my need was again.

"The doctor did not date the Death Certificate. That is why we cannot send it to the County yet for you to pick it up." She said.

"What doctor is that?" I asked.

"The one with Family First Hospice," she replied.

I thanked her and hung up the phone and immediately called Family First. I told them that I was about to go into Probate and needed that Death Certificate. I told them that I had just learned that the doctor did not date the document. I was told they would take care of it as soon as possible.

Later that day UT Southwestern called and said they had faxed the Death Certificate to the County. I called the County and was told it was finally ready to be picked up by me. I drove to the County Courthouse and received copies after I paid for them. Most places like Banks, Life Insurance Companies, and other companies would take Sue's name off the bill with the Death Certificate shown to them. So I worked on the list of things to do before I entered Probate. I Google Probate and found,

"Probate is a legal document. Receipt of probate is the first step in the legal process of administering the estate of a deceased person, resolving all claims and distributing the deceased person's property under a will."

https://www.google.com/#q=Probate

I had to file the Will with the County and wait two weeks for any objections before I could go before a Judge and have her name taken off our bills. I could not sell my house or trade my car until this process was completed. Probate was important to clean up our debt to make it all my responsibility. My Attorney called and said the court wants an eleven hundred dollars filing fee for Probate. I told her never mind that I would keep my money since most everything was not needed to go into Probate due to we did not own that much. Since I found out, my mobile home is like a car and not like a traditional home. Therefore, I did not need to do Probate.

Life changed for me. I did not know what was going to happen next but I assured everyone I was going to take it slow. I sure can mess things up and I knew that was the one thing I did not want to do was mess my life up now. I know how to love now. I know now to stand in faith, I know how to pray now, and I know how to let go and let God take my life and do what He wants done in my life. I am just along for the ride and what a beautiful ride it is walking with God daily. God bless you all who are care givers, you are doing a great work. Stand firm, stay strong, let go and let God move.

Here is a letter dated October 17, 2013 for UT Southwestern Willed Body Program:

"Dear MR. Patterson

On behalf of the University of Texas Southwestern Medical Center at Dallas, I want to express our gratitude for the contributions of Sue Ann Patterson to the Willed Body Program and for your patience during this time. This program is critical to the educational and research missions of the Medical School.

In accordance with our wishes your loved ones cremains are ready to be returned to you. We can either inter the cremains in our Memorial Garden, send them to you by Express US mail or you may contact our office to arrange a time to pick up the cremains at the university. The enclosed forms allow you to tell us your preference. You may mail the form back using the postage paid envelope, or you may email or fax the form to Claudia Yellott. ......"

I mailed back to Claudia Yellott to send Sue' remains in the mail, Seven weeks after Sue's death I was cooking up ten days' worth of food for Travis and I. I got a knock at the door. It was the postal delivery with a box. I signed for the box and then realized the box was Sue's remains left over from her cremation. I knew it was coming but I thought it would not get here this quick. I had asked Claudia Yellott from the Body Willed Program of UT Southwestern if I could know how Sue's body was studied. I received a notice on top of her remains. It was a letter from the Body Willed Program Director.

The letter was dated October 25, 2013. And the letter reads:

"Dear Mr. Patterson, Your wife, Sue Ann Patterson was involved in a course to train Obstetrician/Gynecologist surgeons. On women's health procedures, this training encompasses all areas of women's health and is volatile to their specific area of medicine. The women in our community will benefit from the knowledge the doctors' received form Sue's gift. UT Southwestern Medical Center and our students value the selfless sacrifice made by your family. We now return her to you with humble gratitude and appreciation.

Regards Claudia L. Yellott. Manger UTSW Willed Body Program".

CHAPTER FIFTEEN

The Cost of Caregiving in the Home

There is a huge cost to care giving even in the home. I thought that I could not afford to put Sue into a Nursing home with twenty four seven Skilled Nursing care. I found out I do not know how I even bore the cost of caregiving in the home. On our 1040 A taxes, line 40, 2010 the amount of deductions was $20,507, in 2011 line 40 was $24,679 and in 2012 line 40 was $31,537, and for 2013 this year is $12,400 bringing the total for her care to $89,123. In fact if you add in the part of money that you had to spend in order to meet the line 40 deduction then Sue's care was well over $100,000 in the four years of extreme care. That's a lot of money. The first two and one-half years Sue could take care of herself. 2010 was when I started to administer her care and start of these cost. This last year I was looking at more than $31,537 in cost and bringing home $533 for a month's pay on part-time work.

I say this, to say how Good God truly is. At the end of Sue's life I did not owe a dime on her care. I lost her income and due to God leading me into getting part of her Life Insurance money, the $10,000 before her passing is what has allowed me to go the two months without her income. It allows me to take a month off from life. I needed a month. Really, I need more than a month and it allow me to go do that first month when I went back to work. I did not get paid until the end of the second month. My health is not good. I am so exhausted it almost cost me my life. I now know why Sue started her Living Will early at the end of August instead of October. Sue knew I was dying as well from extreme exhausting. She ended her life early to spare my life!

I'm sure this caregiving experience may have taken years off my life. God is good though. He supplied our needs. He will supply my needs now. For the first time in my Adult Life I am a Single man. That is scary to me; I wanted to grow old with Sue. I do not know why God said No to her healing. I trust God fully.

You see I still was praying for Sue. Her earthy body, I pray that the Holy Spirit stays with the body in a way when these young men and women who were studying Sue's body that they will see treasures in her body, learn from her body and go out and help others with that knowledge. Like I said I did not know why God said No, but I do know that even in death, Sue is reaping blessings in Heaven due to her body blessings other Souls. The ones learning from studying her body to the one who will receive their care in the future. I will love Sue always; I miss her so much already. I have gotten a plot and bought a headstone and on July 4th, her birthday in 2014 I will take her Human remains to where her Mom and Dad lie and burry her remains there with them. I still find myself in my grief still praying for her.

There is a human cost as well! Those who give so much of themselves in caring for their love ones pay such a great cost to their hearts, minds, bodies and Souls. It the most amazing hardship I have ever encounter. Many people out there I am sure will not survive their caregiving service. There are many who are broken down so much that they may never return back to any kind of a Quality of life for themselves. God bless all who give so much of themselves to caregiving their love ones. I am nobody special. I did what God has called every man to do in marriage. To live in good and bad times in sickness and in health, I stayed true to my wedding vowels. I stayed true to my Bride and God will stay true to me. I pray if you are giving care to your love one that you may use this book as a guidance to do as I have done. For I and my family have truly have had one blessed caregiving experience.

CHAPTER SIXTEEN

The Change Needed in Caregiving

Why does the U.S. government allow $89,123 to be spent by one family caregiving in the home? Let me repeat this thought as stated in the introduction.

"Home health care is the fastest growing sector in the health care industry, with an anticipated growth of 66 percent over the next 10 years and with over 7 million patients served each year."
http://ncbi.nlm.nih.gov/books.NBK43619/

I am asking the seventy million families. I am asking two hundred and ten more million Americans who will take care of the seventy million in their homes, Do you have $89,123 to spend on caring for your loved one in the home? I could not believe I spent that much on her care. I ask though, would you help the families of the two hundred and ten million souls who will need your help. The Government is already saying they will not be in the Nursing home. If you gross or have over $2,000 a month than you cannot get help from the United State Government, the State level and most likely the County level as well. Health and Human Services sure did not serve us in any way!

Sue and I did it faithfully. We had God in our midst. That was the only way we made it. I pray when you enter into caring that you have God in your midst as well. I have blessings from caregiving. I am a better man. I have a better walk with the Lord. I have confidence and boldness to go and serve the Lord better now. We need change though.

I could not even get the chance to buy into a Medicaid program. I asked about Survivors Benefits and was informed it was not applicable until you age sixty and even then there are limits. The 2,000 limit gross a month that I could not get past. I tried and got nowhere with Texas or Federal governments. Later in the book you will find that I am making a business plans to help the two hundred and eighty million people. On my web page I plan to have a petition you may sign so we can take millions of signatures to the United States government to make a change. If you spend so much of your income in caregiving why can we not have the Government, the State and County level give an exception to the $2,000 rule for a few years for our families?

I hope the two hundred and ten million people taking care of someone they love in the home will go and sign this petition so we can have change and an exception to the $2,000 a month rule. All I am asking, if I can prove that I do not make $2,000 by a 1040A IRS tax document then I ought to be able to have an exemption to the $2,000 rule. The structure of Health and Human Services is set up right now to penalize you like they did for Sue and I. I would have done better for myself to quit my job, spend my money, sell my home and let the Government take care of me. That's not me though. I stood and fought the Good Fight. I stood in the gap of caregiving so Sue could have a better experience of being cared for.

CHAPTER SEVENTEEN

The application to Caregiving

How you can use this book.

1.) The commitment: without it you will burn out. Caregiving is a choice. Choose so wisely. Some people do not have a successful caregiving experience. You can see in my story the dangers that those APS investigations really became. If your commitment is weak be careful, one can fall into pitfalls of caregiving. Attitude is everything in caregiving. Choose to have a good day. Choose to be strong. Choose to love your loved one. Peace can be there. Get rest, eat and exercise. If you can just do that you will find that caregiving is not so bad after all.

2.) Do the paper work: The Power of Attorneys, the Living Will, the Will. If you do not do the paperwork you leave yourself vulnerable. That day the police were called about the shredding of Sue's mail. I almost went to jail. The female police officer was going for her hand cuffs when I remembered I had done the paper work. The paper work keeps you out of jail. The paper work puts all the burden on you, but, no one can come and take over in the middle of caregiving. The most dangerous caring person is the family member who chooses to stay out of the loop and butts right into the caregiving experience with high stress drama. Take charge of your caregiving experience by doing the paperwork and going with two people that are not in the family to sign off on the paper work with you, your loved one with the Notary. Remember to file it away until the day you need it. Then bring the paper work out and go with it. (Remember I am not a lawyer or Certified Public Account so if you have questions about the paper work then go to them for answers since every caregiving experience is different.)

3.) Research the illness so you know how to care for your loved one better and will know what happens later in the illness. Regardless of the disease whether it is Genetic, Cancer, or an autoimmune disease, Go into caregiving with some knowledge. Remember that the illness affects you all, especially your love one in ways you won't understand. Sue regularly woke me up from much needed sleep for Chap Stick or Puffs. And that was draining. Find out what others are saying about your illness: Google it or Bing it, the illness, in order to find how to better care for your loved one. Life is hard enough make life easier for you.

Care giving becomes much easier if you know how to treat your loved one. There are drugs to find, schedules to make, money to secure, and stress relievers to discover in caregiving. I gave Sue a much better Quality of life by knowing what to do about TIAs, and how to react to slow her bowels moments. I found out how to clean a PICC line that was going into the main artery of her heart. Whenever someone was around who had more knowledge or experience I learned from them as much as I could. Learn what to do in emergencies. All I had to do was grab the 911 packet that was on the wall and take Sue out to the hospital. When I was taking her T-Shirt off and her G-Tube came out. I laid her down on the bed, and grabbed the gauze to put pressure on her stomach and keep her stomach contents from coming out. We whisked off to the Hospital and the nurse said, "That is a good pressure bandage." I went camping each time Sue went to the hospital. I learned what the RN's and Doctors said. I learned a lot on the job when I had to take offenders to the hospital. I would set and watch health care workers work on them and then I went home and put it into practice for Sue. I learned from visiting nurses and intake nurses. Learn how to deal with doctors and pharmacies. Learn how to deal with people in general.

4.) Find ways to vent and take care of yourself otherwise your no good to anyone. Venting is so important. Stress can do lots of bad things to you. There is no room for abuse in caregiving. Be careful of the perception of abuse. I believe that was my problem. Other people would peak into my caregiving world and say, "Oh he must be abusing her."

I would go see a movie or go out to a restaurant and eat a good sit down meal. I bought Sue premium channels to Direct TV. I would find her a good two hour movie and then have time to go to my computer and pray or go just lay down for two hours for rest. I would find moments where she needed rest. I found 70's music with no commercial on Sonic channel. I had such a good hospital bed from Hill-Rom that I made her bed decline to my easy chair. It was like we were lying down together in bed and talking like we did for thirty six years. I would turn the lights out and we would rest for hours. There were times that I enjoyed taking care of Sue. I love her so much even now. I miss her tremendously. This experience will take years to get over. I still need to find ways to vent although that is much easier now. For I know how to vent now.

5.) Learn how Health Insurance works. I teach this to everyone who will listen. Two important words "medically necessary."

The Insurance made a mistake by putting Sue into Custodial Care on everything. When they cut cost, I ran up cost. I learned that Insurance dollars spends like real money. The more I got insurance to pay the more money I did not have to pay. So even though my cost was high it could have been much higher had I not done what I did with them. Insurance is always going to say "No" the 1st time you ask for a benefit. Most people accept no. I would not advise you to take it as far as I did. That was a very long battle. And yet, that battle taught me well. Learn to get the reference numbers to each phone call to the Insurance. If they deny you coverage then Appeal it. They only have a few hours to deal with the Appeal. If a week goes by, call them up and get the reference number and ask where your Appeal is. If you know they should cover it like in Sue's case where a G-Tube was in place and Jeivty was medial necessary. Then go for it. In my case I appealed in house to my Insurance Company, and then appealed it out to the Congressional block. Then the Appeal went back to where the money was with ERS. ERS Company knew it was medically necessary. Learn how to build up supplies: bandages, aspirins, stool softeners, soaps, the list goes on and on. It takes money to meet the needs of caregiving. I went to food pantries so I could have more money for supplies. Travis and I helped the neighbor care for his dying mom while the neighbor was at work. When she passed he gave me her supply of Jeivty. You do not know what that means. There were other days the DME ran me out on Holidays. I called them up and I would say to them, "I bet you ate last weekend!"

They would say,
"Oh I bet you have a plan B."

"My plan B is to go to Walgreens and buy the stuff that puts her into a hospital with an inflamed Pancreas. That's some plan B."

Learn that insurance has a standard to go by Medicare standards. Tell them you want what, *"Medicare allows"* and you will get a whole lot more supplies for the same copay.

6.) Lean how to Work the system. Find out how the system works then work it to your advantage. Believe me I am much more of a go getter now. I am not bashful anymore. I will ask and go for what I need, in the right way of course. Stay within the boundaries. Your best investment is people in the church. They will pray for you. They will help you. They will find money to help you. Money is so tight in caregiving. It cost so much with copays, drug copays and supplies. Find out how much insurance you have and how much your policy pays out. If you do not have insurance go Monday to Social Security and sign up for Medicare/Medicaid. I could have gotten someone paid to come in and care for Sue and Medicaid would have paid for it. I was not eligible for Medicaid. If you gross less than $2,000 a month then you can go and get Medicaid. If you are like me and have some money. It was hard to give up fifty percent of our income. Fifty percent of our take home pay it took the last couple of years. I wanted to have a smooth transition from Marriage to Widower. I did have that smooth transitions. I took off the month of September. I had money to allow me to take that month off. Check into your State to see if it is like Texas when it comes to Hospice. In Texas as long as your love one is consider and on Hospice's care Medicare pays one hundred percent. I sure did not know this but found out it is true. So check into that if your love one is in Hospice and in Medicare.

7.) Be careful not all who say they want to help you truly mean it. Some people want to take advantage of you. I looked out my door one day and saw a car pull up. People piled out of the car like cock roaches. One person came to my door.

"I can get you Medicaid." She said.
"No you can't get me Medicaid." I replied.
"Yes I can." She said.
"I make more than $2,000 a month." I said.
"You are right I cannot bye." She said and left.
Such as the woman I interviewed who wanted me to hire an illegal immigrant. You have to be careful of things like that will get you into trouble.

8.) Faith grows as you go. You will find God like never before in your midst. It is so beautiful how God took care of us. I am a much better man. I am not the same man that for sure. I have changed. In many ways, I am Single now, I hate it. I know how to love now. I not sure if I want to marry again. I do not know my future. I know God will take care of me though. I have a much deeper Faith now. I now see God in beautiful ways. I prayed for Sue while we were married. I prayed for Sue during her illness. I prayed for Sue's body while it was being studied for Science. Then I got her remains back I told myself I cannot pray for her anymore. Then, in my Grief I found that I was praying to God and asking Him to bring Sue to the Throne, and whisper into her ear just how much I miss and love her. I know I have prayed that prayer quite a few times. I am sure some in Heaven now may be wondering why God is Calling Sue to the Throne and why is He whispering into Sue's ear so much!

CHAPTER EIGHTEEN

Thanks to all of you!

I owe a big thank You to many people who helped me with Sue and helped me through these tough years. First I must thank Sue; she was a joy to take care of making us laugh all the time. Thank you to our children, Travis and Jennifer. Travis and Jennifer both helped take care of Sue extensively. Jennifer additionally helped so much on this book re-writing due to my bad grammar. Thank you to those who came into my home from the Home Health groups, the Adult Protection Services to the woman at the doctor office who yelled out to me, "God will bless you for helping her."

I also need to thank all in my job from the Wardens to the Majors, Captains, Sergeants, and Correctional Officers. I must also thank those volunteers who came in to serve at the unit. I thank God for the Navarro County Sherriff department and the Rice police force. You came into my home many times. You busted down my door. You showed me just how powerful the POA is when you were about to throw the cuffs upon me when I shredded Sue's mail.

I thank God for the MS Society. You gave us the one thing that blessed us throughout our experience, the scooter. I thank God for all who prayed for us. I thank all who let me talk. I had so much pain inside that I told anyone who would listen to me my story. I thank God for Hospice. You made the pain so much easier to take in the last days. God bless you all in Hospice, you all do such blessed work. I could not have done this service to Sue without help from others. I thank God for all who work in the Hospitals we went to. Yes I could have gone home and got much needed rest, but I camped out in Sue's hospital room so I would not get behind in her care. Many Nurses, Techs and Doctors blessed us when they came into her room. You showed much skill in compassion. Thank You all who work in this environment, keep up the good work.

I give thanks to God for even the troubles with the Insurance Company put upon us. I know how they work now and can show others how to get around the Insurance mess. I thank God for those who put money into my hand during a hand shake. Those who cared enough for us to tell their Sunday school class to raise money for us. My church, Baylor Baptist who every time I went and asked for money they gave. To the man who ran after me at church and gave me four hundred dollars as I cranked down the window. I thank God for the blessed lady in the back of the church. She hugged me every Sunday and told me she was praying for me. I thank God for the church lady who would come and get my money and list and go and get the stuff in town and bring it back to me. Lord You all do not know how blessed your work was really to me. Thank You my Brothers and Sister in Christ. I thank the church that prayed through all our Living Will days. Those nineteen days were so hard to do. Each day you knew could be Sue's last day on earth. God bless us with blessed Souls who prayed us through the Living Will.

This book is for Jennifer and all who are like her. I remember the day Jennifer sat down after her mom died and said, "I wished someone would have set me down seven years ago and told me what was about to come into our lives." It was amazing to see how Jennifer took the mess I made in dumping out my Soul those few days after Sue's death when I poured out this story. I was a mess and wow did it show up in my story. Jennifer and I took poster size post it notes pads and pasted stories and dates all over her apartment walls. We were trying to pull all the stories in the right time and place that they happened in our lives. It was good to work on this book with Jennifer. I have never written a book before. It took two years to straighten out this story from my messed up life. The re-writes total 24 inches in height. This story is for all the Baby Boomers and their families. There is a big push in the U. S. government that wants us in our homes and not in Nursing homes that the government has to pay for. I showed you all how much it cost Sue and I for her care in our home. It's not cheap.

I hope that you, the reader can see our story as a standard. Thank God if your caregiving is not as bad as ours. God bless you if your experience is worse than our story. I pray that anyone who is considering caregiving may read this story to make life easier for them. I hope you can get things done now even easier than I did.

The one I need to thank the most is God! He was in our midst. Each and every day, each and every hour, each and every minute, though the bad days through the good days. I have never seen God so close to myself before. It is quite beautiful to see God show me what to do and what to say. I was not a brain surgeon, but it was I who looked at the scan before and after the chemo and noticed and told the doctor that the spots were gone from her brain. I am not a Skilled RN. Travis, Jennifer and I did just that, 24/7 Skilled Nursing care in our home to Sue. We are not anything special. God took care of us and is still taking care of us now. I have come out of this experience wounded. I ripped my right knee, my left knee has arthritis. My heart was ripped out and through Share Grief counseling God gave me back my heart. God taught me to live on one paycheck. Now seven months later that just what I am doing living on one paycheck.

When Sue died I did not owe one red cent. God lead me through the valley of death in many beautiful ways. Thank You God for being in our lives. I look forward to moving on. Sue would want me to do just that, move on and go on with life. I also give thanks to my pastor Chet Hensley. You came in late but are dealing with a battle wounded solider of Christ. Thank you for doing Sue's memorial. I need to get healthy again. I need to get emotional healed. I need to get back into serving God. And maybe someday, God will bring someone into my life to bring me back whole again as a man. If I have left you out it's not because I meant too. It just so many people helped us and blessed us it is impossible to remember you all.

I leave you with a prayer:

Lord bless each person who reads our story. May they be blessed seeing You in our midst. May they see a standard to go by for their lives. May they see that they can apply this story in ways that they too can have successful caregiving experience. May they see that this story must be told so others are blessed. This story is for all who are in or are about to go into care giving. Caregiving is a sure, cursed mess that is hard to go through. Let them learn Lord to pray through their struggles. Lord let them learn to take care of themselves. I all most did not make it Lord as you know. You were there all the way Lord. Be with them all the way. Be good to them as You were to us. Empower them so they are blessed and do the things the right way so life is good. You are Good Lord. Thank You for being good to us in the times that Sue went from able body to only a mind. May you bless this book so many other people can find the help they need. Find the way they need to go. Encourage each person who reads and apply this story to their family's lives. So their care giving experience is blessed. I pray you touch each person in this story and all who are our readers. Lord bless my company we are about to open to help the 70 million who will be taken care of in the home and the 210 million who will be helping them and caregiving for them in their individual homes. May You be blessed our Lord and may your Kingdom have a special place for those whom receive and give in the caregiving experience. For we ask in Jesus name, Amen.

CHAPTER NINETEEN

The Letters

This section is for the Power of Attorneys and Letters to Congressmen and women of the United States House and Senate bodies.

These letters follow as:
1. The Power of Attorneys
2. The letter to Congressman Joe Barton
3. The Letters to The House of Representatives and Senate bodies of the United States government.

Our Advance Directives:

1. Durable Family Power of Attorney

I, Sue Patterson appoint John Patterson my husband, my attorney in fact for me and in my name, place, and stead, and for my use and benefit to: act in my capacity to do every act that I may legally do through an attorney in fact, including but not limited to real property transactions; insurance and annuity transactions, claims and litigations, personal and family maintenance, benefits from Social Security, Medicare, Medicaid, or other governmental programs, retirement plan transactions,and tax matters.....

One does not have to do this, but I took this to my county office and had them file it on record. That way anyone that needed to see that this was for sure would find that the county I live in took it as a true record.

2. Durable Family Power of Attorney

I, Sue Patterson appoint: John Patterson as my agent to make any and all health care decisions for me, except to the extent I state otherwise in this document. This durable power of attorney for health care takes effect if I become unable to make my own health care decisions and this fact is certified in writing by my physicians. If the person designated as my agent is unable or unwilling to make health care decisions for me, I designate the flowing persons to serve as my agent to make health care decisions for me as authorized by this document, who serve in the following order: Jenifer Patterson.

3. Living Will

Sue Patterson, having the capacity to make health care decisions, willfully, and voluntarily make known my desire that my dying shall not be artificially prolonged under the circumstances set forth below, and do hereby declare that: If any time I should be diagnosed in writing to be in a terminal conditions by ay the attending physician, or in a permanent unconscious condition by two physicians, and where the applications of life-sustaining treatment would serve only to artificially prolong the process of my dying, I direct that such treatment by withheld or withdrawn, and that I be permitted to die naturally. I understand by injury, disease, or illness that would within reasonable medical judgment cause death within a reasonable period of time in accordance with accepted medical standards, and where the application of life-sustaining treatment would serve only to prolong the process of dying. I further understand in using this form that a permanent unconscious condition means an incurable and irreversible condition in which I am medically assessed within reasonable medical judgment as a having no reasonable probability of recovery from an irreversible coma or a persistent vegetative state. In the absence of my ability to give directions regarding the use of such life-sustaining treatment, it is my intention that this directive shall be honored by my family and physicians (s) as the final expression of my legal right to refuse medical or surgical treatment and I accept the consequences of such refusal. If another person is appointed to make the decisions for me, where through a durable power of attorney or otherwise, I request that the person is guided by this directive and any other clear expressions of my desires.

If I am diagnosed to be in a terminal condition or in a permanent unconscious condition, I do NOT want to have artificially provided nutrition and hydration. I understand the full import of this directive and I am emotionally and mentally capable to make the health care decisions contained in this directive. I understand that before I sign this directive, I can add to or delete from or otherwise change the wording of this directive and that I may add to or delete from this directive at any time and that any changes shall be consistent within Texas state law or federal constitutional law to be legally valid. Sue added to this Living Will: If she chokes again naturally or by food does not want John Patterson to save her life. There is one more PoA that I missed. The Mental PoA. I wonder if I had not missed that PoA if the APS investigations would not have been so many.

These three Advance Directives were signed and notarized on 23rd *day of November 2009. Please note: I gave only the just part of the Advance Directives. I left out personal information of others and parts of the full document. I only wanted you to see the implications that these Advance Directives gave us and the power of these documents in the Court System and Medical World.*

The letter I sent to the Honorable Congressmen Joe Barton.

August 30th, 2010:

To whom it may concern: RE: Sue Patterson,

"Mrs. Patterson is dependent on a feeding tube, and it is medically necessary for her to be fed daily supplements. She is unable to swallow food or liquid. Her only means of sustenance is through a feeding tube. She has been able to gain weight and thrive with the feeding through the feeding tube. She will not be able to live without feeding supplement through the feeding tube," Sincerely, General and Vascular Surgery of Ennis Dr. John Sullivan.

I inquired as to why that letter was not good enough with the Customer Advocate. She placed me on hold. When she returned she informed me that they would accept the letter after all. I continued with caring for my wife, thinking that finally the matter would soon be resolved. I was wrong.

The Kangaroo court really kicked into gear. It started with a letter, dated September 30th, 2010 from insurance company. The letter stated that I needed to provide an itemized bill. I contacted them back and informed the Customer Advocate that they had all of my receipts. I gathered information from them about the itemizations.

I contacted Ennis Medical Supply, at this time, my bill with the company was already up to $2,000, and this bill was solely built up from the acquisitions of Jeivty. I poised my question to them, about whether or not they thought my Insurance Company would actually pay for this Jeivty. With limited options, I had no choice but to continue what we were already doing, and what we were supposed to be on track to do to deal with this situation. I was only going about this, the way that my Insurance Company had agreed that we would deal with this in the first place. Once again, I acquired another months' worth of Jeivty from the Ennis Medical Supply.

In that same pile of mail was another letter from my Insurance Company, which was dated on September 30th, 2010, which claimed that the Date of Service was missing. So I contacted them, informed them, reminded them, that they an already had all of this information, which included the date of service, in the medical file, the medical file of information that I had previously sent. The date of service is June 9th 2010, the date in which the G-Tube was placed into Sue's body. She acknowledged that yes I did indeed sent them a lot of information.

On October 4th, 2010, I received another letter from my insurance company; the letter stated the DME prescription that they had received had gone missing. The following information is what they would require:

Physician's signature
Diagnosis
Length of time DME would be required in days, weeks and months
Whether DME is being rented or purchased

This confused me, I thought my God, what is going on, and surely all of this information is in the medical file. I contacted them yet again.

At this time, I want to inform you, what kind of strain, and stress all of these phone calls to my insurance company have created. My wife's condition status is a total dependency upon someone else to care for her. I had hired an employee, but the employee viewed that her job only lasted during my working hours, as soon as I arrived home from work, she bolted out of the door, she did not even stay long enough for me to change out of my work uniform. The wait period did not even begin until after I entered my personal medical ID number. It would place me on hold in the upward times of two hours at times. Keep in mind; I do not have two hours available to me to sit on hold with the level of care and attention that my wife requires of me. I juggled the phone and my wife, as best as I could.

It turns out that the DME that they were referring to was in reference to a lift chair, a lift chair is not even a part of this case, and one has nothing to do with the other. So after wasting all of this time, it turns out, and this request did not even pertain to the situation.

On October 8th, 2010, I received a letter; this was addressed to Doctor or Provider. I did not understand this letter, so I contacted a customer advocate of my insurance company to get clarification. I was informed that the letter was an attempt by a provider for the purpose of checking out my insurance.

Then I received a letter which was dated October 13th 2010. It was from the company whom supplies the money, my insurance company were administers only to my policy. My Insurance Company logo was on it, and a check for $128.70 was inside of it. I compared this check amount, to my receipts, decided that this was only a small part of my actual claim. It did not cover all the supplements I bought out of my pocket with Walgreen's, let alone all the Jeivty that had been acquired from the Ennis Medical Supply. So I contacted the office of my insurance company and waited on hold yet again for two hours. Once I got a hold of a customer advocate, I requested to speak with a supervisor. The supervisor, at the Dallas office, stated that the amount of $128.70 was all that they were going to pay for. She stated that they refused to pay for anything else.

I decided that this had gone on long enough. I contacted my Attorney Jean DeWald. Jean suggested that my insurance company should have a process that they could set up, internally, in order to challenge this in house with an appeal.

A couple days later I contacted the Dallas office and requested that I wanted to start the process of an appeal, the cause for the appeal was to find out why they were refusing to pay for the nutritional supplements. They transferred me to another office where we were able to start the appeal process. They took all the information from me and the reasons why I was requesting the appeal.

On February 19th, 2011, I received another letter from my Insurance Company stating they required an itemized bill. I thought here we go again; we have already been through this once before. I contacted the customer advocate again, waiting another two hours on the phone to do so.

By this time, I am tired, I am worn out, and I have been care giving for my wife since March 2007. Since the placement of the G-Tube, the duties required for care giving had greatly increased. Ultimately my wife suffers from a breakdown of the Central Nervous System, but so far we do not know the cause for this, or what is required in order to fix it. It is an ongoing medical investigation. As of this date, Doctor or Test knows what is the real cause of the CNS breaking down in Sue's body is. I continue to persist and persevere. I am working a full time job outside of the home, I am working a full time job inside of the home, I am working a full time job of running a small business in order to have an employee to care for my wife while I am at work, and I am working a full time job in order to gather, record, present, all the medical documentation not only for tax purposes, but also for records and requests from my Insurance Company of Dallas. From 3 A.M, to 4 A.M. I care for my wife, at 4:30 A.M I am on the road driving to work.

One night, I set out to call the Dallas office, I was tired, I was not aware that I was calling after 7 P.M., and I did not know that after 7 P.M., all calls are routed to Albuquerque, New Mexico office of my insurance company. I was shocked! In a few minutes I had a customer advocate. I sat there for another two hours listening to this man name Gary apologizing to me for my inconveniences that the company he represents has caused. How my insurance company had dropped the ball over and over with their dealing with us. I told him exactly what all I have gone through while dealing with their Dallas office. He acknowledged that the company had did us wrong.

I waited a couple of days, and then I contacted Gary, to check up on the status of my appeal. He said something about UT Southwestern. Later I got to thinking about that call, over the course of a week, and I decided that I needed to call Gary back up. We talked about the UT Southwestern in further detail. He acknowledged that the appeal was for my UT Southwestern Anesthesiology bill. I informed him, that's not even what my appeal was for. I reminded Gary, that my appeal was for an unpaid claim involving my unpaid itemizes receipts and not anything else. Gary requested that I gather all of my information about the receipts that I have, and fax them directly to him. He asked that on the cover sheet that I put as the following:

Fax 505-962-****

Attention Gary 305*

Membership number, my personal number for insurance company

John Patterson 903-602-****

I AM APPEALING THE NON-REMIMBURSMENT OF RECIPTS

Attach is the copy of the original receipts.

There is a night and day difference between the Albuquerque office and the Dallas office.

Gary contacted me; evidently some of the receipts were not that good for imaging, so he and other technicians black marked what was bad on the fax and then sent it in for imaging. Gary and I began conversing, and we talked several things out. He gave me respect as a person. He understood the position I was in involving with the care of my wife. He even took time to listen to me about the CNS breakdown.

Then one day I came across this letter. The letter provided me with information about the rights of an Appeal. It is titled important updates. In this letter are states as follows:

You must be notified of urgent care claims benefit determination no later than 25 hours after the receipt of your claim, unless you fail to provide sufficient information. You will be notified of the missing information and will have no less than 48 hours after the missing information is received…..We will provide you with any new or additional evidence or rational and any other information and documents used in the adverse benefit determination so you have a reasonable opportunity to respond before a final decision is made.

I contacted Gary and informed him of this information that is in writing from my insurance company. Reading this information, it acknowledges that you have violated our rights to an appeal. This started June 9th 2010. Today is April 20th 2011, and nothing has been resolved on this matter. Well when I communicated this to Gary I requested to speak with his supervisor. His supervisor in Albuquerque contacted me. Her name is Chris; she gave me her personal cell number.

Some things have changed, but not many, since I stated that my insurance company had violated our rights to an appeal. No longer does it take two hours to get through on the Dallas office. I was setting at home one day in March of 2011 when the phone rang. I answered the call; it was Chris the supervisor and she requested to speak with Dr. John Sullivan. I informed her that I was not Dr. Sullivan but that I was in fact John Patterson.

Chris recognized my name a stated that she was trying to get a hold of Dr. Sullivan for the diagnosed code so that she could begin my claim. I informed her that I would get the number for her. I hung up the phone with her and contacted Dr. Ennis Care Center.

I asked the person working if Dr. John Sullivan was on call tonight? She acknowledged that he was. I asked if she would contact Dr. Sullivan and request him to call me at home over a question with the insurance company. She informed me that the doctors were not on call to answer questions that are based about insurance. I looked at my wife, she had been picking her nose with a tissue, and on that tissue were spots of blood, so I told the woman I was speaking with her to inform the doctor that my wife had a nose bleed.

An hour later Dr. John Sullivan contacted me, I ask him what the diagnose code was the he used on the placement of my wife's G-Tube. He said he was not aware of codes, but the name of the diagnoses is Dysphagia. I had him spell the word out for me. We also discussed the nose bleed. Dr. Sullivan said to put pressure on the bridge of the nose to stop the bleeding. I Google Dysphagia and found more information on swallowing difficulties.

This was what Dallas should have asked for a long time ago. And the first thing they should have been asking for from me back in August of 2010. That night I called Chris in Albuquerque, I got her voicemail, and I left a voice mail, with the name of the reason for the placement of the G-Tube and spelled the word as well for her. Then I contacted a customer advocate in Albuquerque, she was very pleasant to speak with. She stated she would send everything we spoke about to Gary in the form of an email; I specifically made sure she understood to include the diagnoses and the explanation of what that diagnoses meant. I told the customer advocate, that the level of service I have received from the New Mexico office; make me want to move to New Mexico.

I contacted Gary once again to inform him about this new tactic that Dallas is using on me. Gary warned me that I was going to receive another letter dated March 22nd 2011 was coming. It was yet again, another request, for an itemized bill.

The following are reference numbers to conversations that I have had with the office of my insurance company in Dallas and in Albuquerque most of the conversations listed are from Albuquerque. I have requested my insurance company to give me a printed out copy of these conversations that these reference numbers refer to, but my insurance company has denied that to me as well. All of these reference numbers involved everything that I have already stated for you previously in this letter. The reference numbers are as follow:

1-25*295*079
1-25*295*079
1-261*8361*8
1-2*16*767*3
1-*62*944*56

Here are my points:
1). Not all things that have been labeled as Custodial Care are actually Custodial Care items, some things are medical necessities.
2). When they surgically inserted the G-Tube into my wife, I received and RX for Jeivty later, they should not have said, "NO" to the request to supply nutritional supplement, but rather they should had said, yes. This procedure was a necessity to prevent death by means of starvation. The inflamed panaceas did not have to happen, along with the 68 hours of hospitalization and the dollars that were spent if they had simply not said no the first-time I tried to get Jeivty.
3). The Failure of the Dallas office to listen, and to act, is beyond disappointing. I was transferred all over their office internally; I spoke again and again to different representatives of that office. I even started the appeal process in this office. How they managed to confuse the

actual problem with a bill from UT Southwestern is beyond my comprehensions. I bet if I took the time and investigated the UT Southwestern bill that it would reflect as already paid for.

4). The incompetence of Dallas to take the appeal, misfile the appeal, mislabel the appeal, and then allowing the appeal to just sit on a table for months, because they could not take the time to bother themselves with it, and not looking at it again until I sent that fax to Albuquerque in March of 2011. I learned this information from Gary; he informed me that the appeal had just lain on a table in an office for the last several months.

5). The letters, the run around, and the phone calls cost me precious time. Time that I just do not have to be wasting, that never should have taken this time at all. I have a full time job, I also have a full time job as a caregiver, a full time job as an employer, and a full time job making/filing paperwork, and keeping track of medical charts, receipts, bills paid, bill that need to be paid, records, taxes, my employee, data entry, and everything else that I have to do, that has added needed, unwanted and unwarranted stress. My time is precious.

6). I feel the customer advocate program is set up to defeat the purpose of obtaining help in Dallas. I stand up for my rights, and the rights of others. I am sure most people would have given up and dropped this process in defeat a long time ago.

7). The office of my insurance company showed nothing but incompetence, and an inept ability to perform their job on a basic level. They not only dropped the ball, but they threw the ball away.

8). This is a poor way to attempt to operate a business. The $128.70, a partial payment, is not by policy covered 80%

of coverage, but it does show an intent to pay. I cannot fathom why they chose to drag this out, why they chose to allow the Ennis Medical Supply bill to get up to $2,000 before they started to pay. Not paying the Jeivty at 80% is not within their policy guidelines. Also they do not want to pay for the supplements that I purchased at Walgreen's, since they were bought over the counter. The only reason why the supplements where purchased over the counter was because they refused to pay for the original request of the payment at the Ennis Medical Supply. I was forced to obtain the supplement as I could, when I could, as my pay allowed when this first began. They said, "No" June 9th, 2010. This is what created this situation. It was not my original choice to buy supplement over the counter, or my original intent.

9). The Medical file, which I purchased with cash out of my pocket, to obtain for them. After I copied it, I sent their copy to my Insurance Company in their Dallas office. It has all of her medical information, which included the diagnoses, with which I have highlighted in blue where it is mentioned ten times that her diagnoses is Dysphagia as listed and sated above. The level of incompetence, laziness, ineptness, under qualified staff, untrained staff, lack of caring, whatever the reason is, and the Dallas office is below any acceptable level of standards.

10).Ten months later, an issue that should have been resolved with 24 to 48 hours, is still left unresolved. It is my belief that my insurance company has violated our RIGHTS to an Appeal, the only question is, were these rights violated belatedly, intentionally, or by ineptness to perform their job on a basic level. Was it done purposely, with intent, or by incompetence, regardless of the reason, the matter of the situation is regardless of the reason any excuse in unacceptable.

Thank you for your time,

John Patterson

John Patterson

Letters I sent to House and Senate of the U.S Congressman

Dear Honorable United States Senator,

Hi, my name is John Patterson, I am looking for help. My wife Sue and I have been married 36 years. In March of 2007, Sue was diagnosed as having two frontal lobe strokes by neurologists. I prayed to God and ask Him to heal her. The strokes and what came with it lifted and went away in her body. I praised God and went on with our lives.

Then the worst fears were realized. She declined rapidly. She appears to have symptoms that resemble Parkinson's, MD, Multiple Sclerosis. She would fall down, a lot. Much money and years have been spent trying to find out simple diagnoses. One day that I rushed a critical MRI for her. I took her to UT Southwestern in Dallas.....and she would not lie upon the table she was so badly bruised from her falls. Then we found another symptom in her life. CASDIAL, CASDIAL is lined up to a "T" to her illness. She has two test performed and found that she was negative on both of them. There is no false positive for this genetic disorder, there are false negatives. Even more symptoms came into her life. In all 11 illnesses were ruled out. She has legions upon her neck area. These legions are not like the MS legions for these legions are the exact copy of one another. She has spots on her brain. These spots have changed her personality. What she hated she loved and what she loves she hated. She put me into three Adult Protective investigations; the hospital lab put me into one investigation. All of these investigations were concluded that I had not abused her.

We went and did Durable Power of Attorneys, both health and medical. We agreed that her body would be willed to UT Southwestern for study for one year then after the study they will cremate her and give her back to me. Whatever this illness is, I would not wish it on anyone to have it including my worst enemy.

My first employee lasted 3 months before she could not do the job. Another employee was hired after that. She seemed fine, but I think the stress of the situation just overcame her; she left on her own accord. Our Son Travis is now with us. He has been here over a year helping us. About 18months ago Sue went from an independent woman to a total dependent woman. She can do nothing for herself.

I realized she was starving to death; I made a phone call to a surgeon and scheduled an appointment. We went, he says to her wait, he left the room came back and said we are going to do her labs here, and then meet me at the surgery center in an hour. We did and this surgeon placed a feeding tube into her stomach wall. I asked the surgeon what now? He gave me a script for Jeivty 1.2 and said go get this at the DME store. I took Sue home then, later went to the medical store supply, gave them my insurance information, the insurance denied me coverage.

I did what I had to do; I went to a retail store and purchased strawberry and chocolate nutritional drinks. I started pouring in, five cans a day. There months later I had to take Sue to the hospital. The shakes had inflamed her Pancreas. I had to starve her for three days to calm down the Pancreas. Then the Nutritional lady came into the room and said we needed Jeivty 1.2 not the brand we were using. We called the insurance company and they approved her five cans a day of Jeivty 1.2.

I asked them to pay for the last 3 months prior to the hospital stay. I sent in all the paper work and they denied the claim.

I have been in constant battles with my Insurance Company to the point that I brought in Honorable Joe Barton into the situation. He is my local congressman. He did an insurance inquiry. We finally learned that my insurance company had thrown my request into The Company who supplied the money. I work for the Texas Department of Criminal Justice in the capacity of a corrections officer. This Company told me, "Your letter spurred us into actions."

They sent it back to my Insurance Company and told them to pay me, which my insurance company finally did so.

I have learned some things during this hardship. In my case I have learned 11 illnesses only to find that any one of them may crop up and have symptoms at any time and last for a few minutes, a few hours, a few days or even months. I have learned to take care of myself. The better I take care of myself the better care I can give. I have learned to treat this as a business and because I have employees have set it up as a business so that I can keep working outside of the home. I have learned to be on call 24/7. I have learned that doctors are on call so use that resources and contact them. I have learned that no one can help you if you don't ask. I have learned to call RN Service from my insurance card. I have to do things I never thought I would ever do in my life. I have learned to take complete care of my loved one for she is totally dependent on someone one else to help her do her daily task of living. I have learned to fight for her. I have learned not to wait, see any sign of infections and do something about it immediately before the infection gets any worse. I have learned not to sweat the small stuff. I have learned I do not know it all. I have learned you have to fight the insurance company; their first response is always No, so ask again. I have learned to give it to God in prayer. I have learned knowledge about the care giving process and many aspects of it. So I try to help others however I can, even if it's just with advice.

I have had several social workers come into my house. They say, "If anyone needs to be on Medicaid it is your wife, but you make too much money!" I am penalized because I work. My Insurance Company says she "Custodial Care." Texas Department Assistive and Rehabilitation Services gave us a ramp, a nice ramp. This is the one and only time that a government agency did anything for us; then they heard Custodial care and did nothing else. DARS called me up one day to inform me Sue had moved up on the waiting list. You can get your doctor co-pays and RX copays paid up to $1,000 a month. Outstanding! Sadly, I started a 30 hour research project for this program, sat there with this lady from DARS with 50 pages that they requested me to obtain for them, but we were unable to get past page two, Income. I cannot place my wife in an assisted living home, because she is 52 and not 62. We attempted the Nursing home route, we visited four locations, but all of them require a minimum $150 a day, 24/7 skilled nursing care due to her dependence and they will not take our insurance, so after everything is said and done and added up, you're looking at almost to more money a month than we could afford. Our income is less than $4,000 a month. So we are left to just do the best we can with what we have.

I had to become an employer and pay for employees out of the money we bring home. I pay for a half million dollars' worth of workman's comp policy so that no one can sue us if they get hurt while taking care of Sue. Sue is a full body lift. She cannot do anything for herself. On a good day she can put Chap Stick up to her mouth, but most of the time she's not able to even do that.

We discussed with the neurologist what our options were; they decided we should attempt experimental chemo that they have been seeing some success with, with other neurological patients. She was near death and the doctor said that this is our only option. It took 4 months to argue with the insurance company to approve it because she doesn't have cancer. Then it took a year for an urologist to figure out why she was getting urinary tract infections. We found that she was retaining urine and that was what was creating the issues and why she was having constant chronic infections.

We went to Ashton Building hospital in Dallas to do the chemo. The results were amazing! Everyone could see that his was affecting her in a positive way. The chemo we use was Methotrexate, a drug that went generic and then the EPA shut down the only lab that was making it in the United States. So we got a glimpse of hope, and then had it stripped from us. We were supposed to get our third chemo treatment in March of 2012, but the doctor said,

I'm sorry, but we cannot get Methotrexate for another 6 months at least!" Heartbreaking news, to say the least, The next six months of her even surviving is bleak, to say the least, without the Methotrexate.

I looked at an MRI of her brain before chemo and a MRI after chemo. I saw that the white spots on her brain were diminished. I emailed the doctor and said, "What say you?" Seven days later the doctor emailed me back and said, "The enhancements are gone." The doctor put her on Cell Cept; she is on a liquid form of Methotrexate. She is taking 2,000 ml of Cell Cept a day. I give it to her a 3 A.M. and at 7 P.M. Every day I get up a 3 A.M. take care of her and for an hour to an hour and 1/2 then drive to work.

I work full time, I care give full time, I work full time doing paperwork because I have to treat this as a business. This has not been easy for any of us. Sue lives on. She can set up in a chair or lay in a bed. She has one finger out of ten that she can use to peck out short sentences to communicate to us on a laptop, or her desktop computer. Her world is small now. I am forever grateful for my Son Travis my daughter Jennifer's help. Without them I could not do this for Sue.

We are trying to get help anywhere we can. I pay 71% of our adjusted gross income to take care of Sue. Why can I not get a waiver from *Medicaid*? Why is there not a way to get some form of help? As I write this letter I am in appeal with *Medicaid*. I am appealing that, yes I make too much money, but look at what I pay out. It took $24,000 out of my pocket for her healthcare needs for my wife in 2011! That is a lot of money. I challenge anyone to let me have $24,000 out your hard earned money. You would not do it willingly. I do this because I love my wife. Why not if one can prove with IRS tax return that one pays so much out in medical that an exception to the $2,000 rule be possible? Why can we not make a change in that $2,000 rule?

Here is some quotes from an 83 page report on caregiving in the U.S:

People who care for adult family members or friends fulfill an important role not only for the people they assist, but for society as a whole. While this care is unpaid, its value has been estimated at 257 billion dollars annually.

Although care giver's make many contributions, being a care giver may take a personal toll.

Arno, P. S. Economic Value of Informal Caregiving.

We estimate there are 44.4 million American care givers (21% of the Adult population. Age 18 and older that provide unpaid care to an adult age 18 or older, the care givers are present in an estimated 22.9 million households, 21% of US households).

The actual numerical estimate of care giver's is 44,442,800

The actual numerical estimate of care giving households 22,901,800

For more information for this report go to http://www.caregiving.org/data/04finalreport.pdf

Therefore, Honorable US Senator, I am one out of millions. We need help. Those whom are burden, spending, dealing, toiling with those whom they love need a helping hand at times. I am seeking help not just for myself, but for everyone! There needs to be a change, we need help, you were elected to be a voice of the people, and the people who are suffering in this injustice need you now more than ever!

There are so many things, that we as care giver's needs, just as hospital beds in the home. Lifts, wheel chairs, so many things, and the insurance company have labeled all of these things to be Custodial Care. Custodial Care is 100% paid out of my pocket! It's a need, these are needs we need help with our needs.

I am including 2010 and 2011 tax returns. I will also give you the totals of the first 4 months of this year. Please just take a little bit of your time to read and understand what I am saying to you! We need a little help. Will you please help us?

Thank you for your time,

John Patterson

About the Author

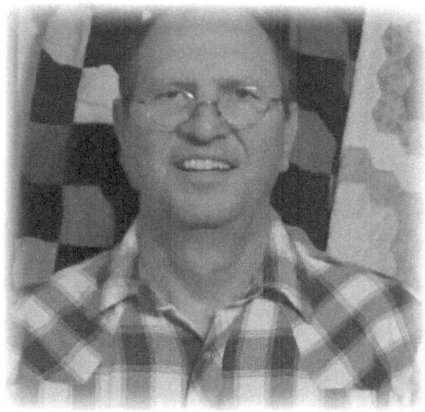

John Patterson is a changed man. He is more of a man now after having gone through this precious time with Sue. He grew up poor and humbled. The years of marriage with Sue were a blessing beyond measure. He was first person in his family to go to College and graduate with a Bachelor of Arts from Southwest Baptist University. He currently works for the State of Texas. He still attends church regularly and is always willing to help anyone in need that he comes in contact with.

He wrote this book for his daughter Jennifer, his son Travis, those in or entering into the caregiving field, and the Baby Boomer generation and their individually family members and freinds. He hopes all who reads this book discovers a better way to apply caregiving through his experience. He hopes that all who read this book will be able to see God present and among us, no matter the circumstances that we are faced with in this life. He believes that this book has the ability to change lives, and change them for the better.

His life goal is to find a way to change policies within the United States Congress, State regulations, any way to change the view point to the current laws where the $2,000 rule is currently applied. He wants to see an exception to this rule so that your family does not have to pay out thousands of dollars out of your budget like we had to do.

Book Reviews before sending into publisher:

Pastor Chet said, "There is lot of material in such short period of time."

Hospice RN Vick she said, "I could not put your book down, and I was so interested. It was like you put my feelings on paper. I really could feel how you felt. I have such a new respect for you, I'm really impressed."

Hospice Brenda said, "Amazing Story!! I love it. You did a great job! Everything is in such detail. I love the page that has "the board" on it. Brought back lots of memories!!

Other Works by this Author

How to Set Up Caregiving In the Home
Volume 2
From the Book, Caregiving: Our Labor of Love book series.
By: John Patterson
COPYRIGHT 2016 by JOHN PATTERSON.

The book provides the details and presents the knowledge of how a family can set up caregiving in their home. It begins with what is called the 911 packet. This packet takes critical information and easily presents it in one place. You take this packet with you to your doctor or hospital visits. The hospital will then take this packet and scan it into their system. The Information will be present in their system now and the Doctors, Pharmacists, RN's or others can easily see what is happening with the patient. The hospital staff will be able to see the details of the patient such as weight, age, height, allergies, and drugs. Drugs are listed with name, strength and how many times a day. The patient receives optimal care, less money is expended, and the hospital does not have to waste time/money trying to collect the information that you have already presented them with. The hospital will take this 911 packet and incorporate it into their plan for your love one.

This book will carefully present to you on how to properly make and maintain a budget. Included is a gas book: easily keep track of each time you fill up your gas tank by recording the date, mileage at the time up fill up, number of gallons used to fill the car, and the price per gallon. Using this data that you gathered over the course of a month, you will be able to see how many gallons of gas you used. Using this information with the price you paid at the pump you'll then be able to budget for the next month on you gas expenditures. You'll also be able to utilize this information to uncover how many miles per gallon your vehicle is getting. Each month you'll know in advance what your gas expense should be, and if suddenly the mile per gallon drops one month, then you'll know it's time to perform some maintenance on your car. Maintaining the car will also help reduce unwanted expenses.

This book will teach you how to utilize the power of Attorney and help you understand its importance. It's the actual wording from the Department of Aging and Disability Services of Texas.

Please note I am not an Attorney so I will not be advising you on these directives. Also the information will vary from state to state. My experience in dealing with them was in relation to the state of Texas. Any legal questions that you have should be followed up with your legal counsel. I can only stress the importance of having a Power of Attorney. I can show you what it looks like within the book.

The book shows you how to take you receipts and track against the itemized deductions on line 40 of 1040A. When you start adding up receipts that are allowed, then you can minus them off of your taxes and get that money back from your taxes.

The book will show you some common practices if you have a primary and secondary insurance. By watching the bills when they come in, you can catch a practice that puts secondary insurance first and primary insurance second. This practice could end up costing you thousands of dollars if you do not catch it. All you have to do is call them and inform them who is your primary and who is your secondary. Doing this may save you thousands of dollars on insurance cost.

This book will teach you how to find financial assistance. There is money out there to help you in this time of need. I will show you where to go. I cannot guarantee you will receive the help, but there are some real possibilities available out there. I touch on Hospice only to show you how to get Hospice paid 100%. I also will show you in this book how to set up a business with the IRS to bring in an employee into your home. You may not need to do this, but the information is here for you just in case. Some people may need this kind of help in order to maintain their current career in order to keep affordable insurance that they already have.

(One may buy this book by writing to John Patterson, Caregiving A Labor of Love, LLC,P. O. Box 22, Rice TX 75155. The price is $15 plus S& H for a total of $22.00. We accept checks, money orders or credit cards.)

Caregiving: Continues Care
Volume 3
This book will be out early 2017. In this book I will take you from Home Set Up into Continues Care. This kind of Care builds from easy to tremulously hard. It will show you where you are going in caregiving. It will show you the painful part of watching your love one fade. It will deal with the daily grind, the sleeping with one ear open, the hit the floor running when you get out of bed. It will show you how to do 24 hour 365 days a year care. Continues care is all the way until the passing of a love one. It is

tough to say the least. I will show you how to do it better and find and make blessed memories.

Caregiving: Life After When Your World is Turned Upside Down
Volume 4

This book will show you what is needed right after the passing of a love one. I will show you the process of starting over. I will share with you a fantastic Greif counseling service at no cost to you. I will show you to take it easy the first two years. There are traps out there waiting for you to come along while you are so down in life. Life is beautiful and this book will help you get back to that beautiful life that you had before you started the caregiving process. This book will be out in the Spring/Fall of 2018.

Helpful Links

National Alliance for Caregivers: http://www.caregiving.org/
The American Heart Association: http://heart.org/
The National MS Society: http://www.nationalmssociety.org/
American Cancer Society: http://www.cancer.org/
The National Parkinson Society: http://www.parkinson.org/
American Lung Association: http://www.lung.org/
Medicare: http://www.medicare.gov/
The United House of Representatives: http://www.house.gov/representatives/find/
The United States Senate: http://www.senate.gov/general/contact_information/senators_cfm.cfm
Find your state representatives: http://openstates.org/find_your_legislator/
Internal Revenue Services. http://www.irs.gov/
Google: The Workforce Commission for your State Texas Example: http://www.twc.state.tx.us/
Need Prayer Requests Visit Guide Posts: http://www.guideposts.org/faith-in-daily-life
Google: Department on Aging and Disability Services Texas Example: http://www.dads.state.tx.us/
Grief Share: http://www.griefshare.org/

Coming soon to the Web

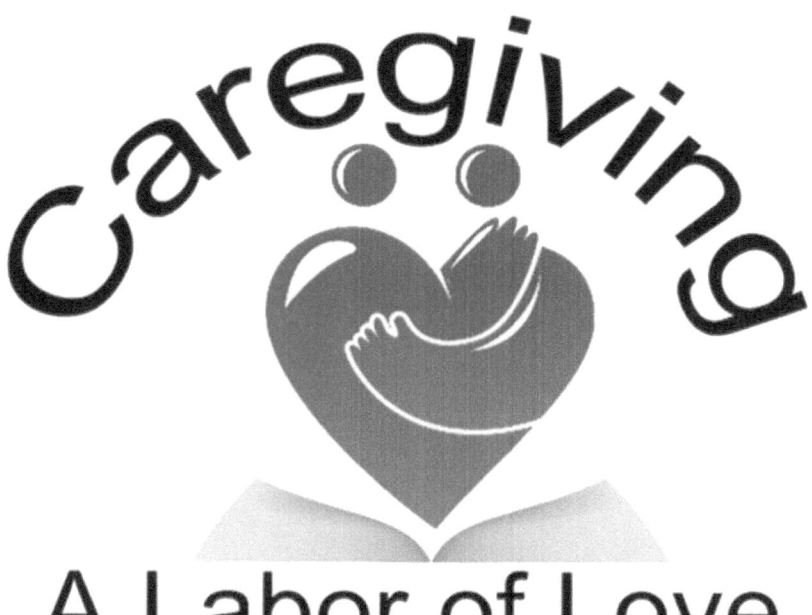

Caregiving
A Labor of Love

www.ingramcontent.com/pod-product-compliance
Lightning Source LLC
Chambersburg PA
CBHW032007170526
45157CB00002B/590